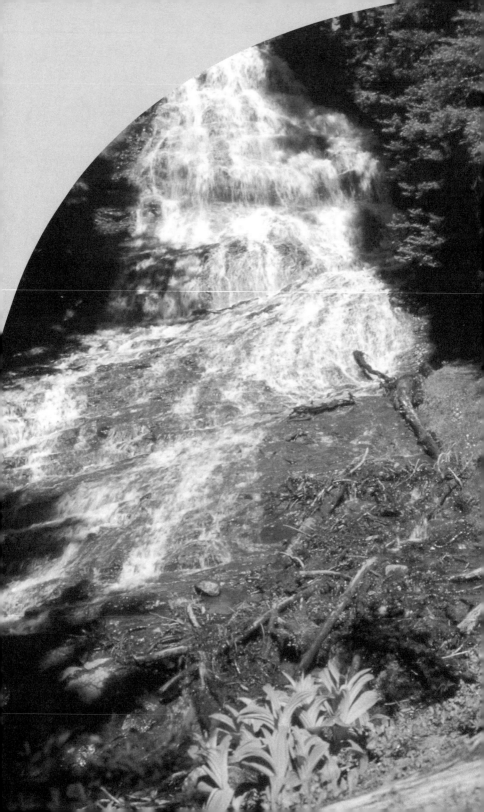

ONE NIGHT WILDERNESS
PORTLAND

Quick & convenient backpacking getaways
within three hours of the city

Douglas Lorain

WITHDRAWN

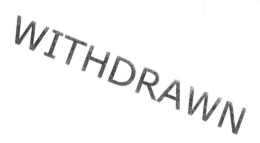 **WILDERNESS PRESS** ... *on the trail since 1967*

BERKELEY, CA

One Night Wilderness: Portland: Quick & convenient backpacking getaways within three hours of the city

1st EDITION 2009
   2nd printing August 2009

Copyright © 2009 by Douglas Lorain

All photos and maps copyright © 2009 by Douglas Lorain (except photo on p. 234)
Cover design: Larry B. Van Dyke
Book design: Lisa Pletka
Book editor: Marc Lecard

ISBN 978-0-89997-463-7

Manufactured in the United States of America

Published by: **Wilderness Press**
               1345 8th Street
               Berkeley, CA 94710
               (800) 443-7227; FAX (510) 558-1696
               info@wildernesspress.com
               www.wildernesspress.com

Visit our website for a complete listing of our books and for ordering information.

Cover photos: Three Fingered Jack from the Pacific Crest Trail, Mount Jefferson
                   Wilderness (Trip 62) *(front);* Mt. Hood above Mt. Hood Meadows
                   (Trip 41) *(back)*
Frontispiece: Umbrella Falls, Mount Hood National Forest (Trip 41)

"Having a landscape to oneself is an exclusive pleasure. Many of us stumble upon this by surprise. Suddenly it is there—unshared, solitary. One may well experience a reckless moment of freedom, a penetrating moment of understanding. A meaning that was elusive is suddenly clear."

—*Margaret Owings,*
artist and conservationist

Acknowledgments

As always, the help of many people made this book possible. Special thanks go to the following persons:

For her love, her encouragement, and especially her forbearance in allowing me to spend so much time on the trail (sadly) away from her loving arms, I especially wish to thank my wife, Becky Lovejoy.

I would also like to thank my nephews, Rossin and Kamron Ebrahimi, and Drew Bush, who enthusiastically helped me experience the joys of introducing a youngster to backpacking (and stuffing my face with huckleberries) on their first overnight trips into the wilderness.

My great appreciation goes to all the many people at Wilderness Press whose talent and hard work were invaluable in making this book both readable and attractive, but who (unfairly) don't get the glory of having their names on the cover. On this project I especially want to point out the assistance of Marc Lecard, Lisa Pletka, and Laura Shauger.

Finally, I would like to thank the following individuals at the various land agencies for taking the time to review hikes in their area and provide helpful input: Steve Andringa, Bryan Bell, Susan Graham, Edan Lira, Jon Nakae, Jacquelyn Oakes, Jim Thornton, Geoff Walker, and Macy Yates.

Preface

Fortune has smiled on outdoor lovers in the Portland metropolitan area. Within a short drive from their homes, hikers face an almost unbelievable array of options. They can choose to walk through massive old-growth forests or to visit any of several hundred waterfalls. They can climb across massive glaciers or traipse through wildflower-covered mountain meadows. They can beachcomb on surf-pounded sand or explore semi-desert canyonlands filled with the aroma of sagebrush. Only one or two other cities in the country can boast such a wide assortment of opportunities so close at hand.

Many, even most, of these wonders are accessible to dayhikers. But as thousands of pedestrians have discovered over the years, to appreciate fully the charms and wonders of the wilderness, nothing compares to packing in your gear and spending the night. The outdoor experience is infinitely richer, more exhilarating, and certainly more memorable if you extend your stay, enjoying a place where the stars outshine the streetlights, where the hooting of owls and the howling of coyotes replaces the honking of horns and the shriek of sirens, and where crowded cityscapes, although closer than you'd think, seem to be a million miles away.

This book is designed for two groups of people: those who already know the pleasures and rejuvenating qualities of spending a night in the wilderness; and those who hope to soon join that club. The goal is to provide the first guide to all the best one- (and a few two-) night hikes within a three-hour drive of Portland. There are trips here for all ability levels, from short and easy strolls suitable for backpackers of any age, to extended trips of 20 miles or more that will test even the fittest hiker. What they all have in common is a close proximity to Portland, terrific scenery, and inviting campsites that make them suitable for weekend trips.

While researching this guide, I hiked every trip in this book at least once and most of them numerous times. However, roads and trails constantly change as new routes are built, old trails are abandoned, and floods and landslides obliterate existing routes. Your comments on recent developments or changes for future editions are always welcome. Please write to me in care of Wilderness Press at info@wildernesspress.com.

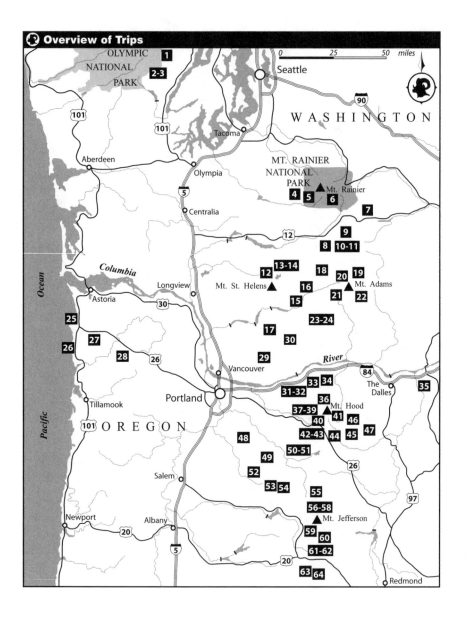

Overview of Trips

Contents

Summary of Featured Trips

EASY HIKES	Scenery	Difficulty	Solitude	Miles	Elev. Gain	Trail Use
1 Duckabush River Trail (first camp)	5	2	6	4.4	900	kids
3 Lower Lena Lake	6	4	2	6.2	1350	kids
8 Cispus Point	7	3	9	5.6	1400	kids, dogs
9 Packwood Lake	6	3	2	9	300	kids
15 Lewis River Trail	5	2	6	5.2	200	kids, dogs
16 Quartz Creek	5	3	8	9.2	750	kids, dogs
17 Siouxon Creek	7	2	4	7.6	700	kids, dogs
23 Lemei and Blue Lakes Loop	7	4	5	12.3	1800	kids, dogs
25 Tillamook Head (south)	6	4	4	3	820	
27 Soapstone Lake	5	1	9	2.4	250	kids, dogs
28 North Fork Salmonberry River	5	2	9	4.2	840	kids, dogs
29 Silver Star Mountain (north)	8	4	6	5.6	1700	kids, dogs
30 Soda Peaks Lake	6	4	7	4.6	1300	kids, dogs
32 Eagle Creek (Tenas Camp)	9	3	2	8	750	
34 North Lake	6	1	6	1.6	190	kids, dogs
35 Lower Deschutes River Canyon	7	4	5	7.3	820	kids, dogs
37 Ramona Falls	6	4	5	7	1100	kids, dogs
41 Elk Meadows	7	4	5	6.6	1250	kids, dogs
42 Salmon River Trail (lower)	6	1	6	4	250	kids, dogs
43 Veda Lake	5	3	8	2.8	750	kids, dogs
44 Lower Twin Lake	5	2	4	4	700	kids, dogs
45 Boulder Lake	6	1	7	0.6	200	kids, dogs
47 Badger Creek	5	2	7	5.8	450	kids, dogs
48 Memaloose Lake	5	2	6	2.8	700	kids, dogs
50 Shining Lake	7	3	6	8.8	800	kids, dogs
51 Shellrock Lake	7	1	4	1.4	200	kids, dogs
53 Pansy Lake	6	1	5	2.2	400	kids, dogs
55 Olallie Lake Scenic Area Loop	7	3	5	9.1	1200	kids, dogs
57 Firecamp Lakes	6	2	4	2.4	640	kids, dogs
59 Pamelia Lake	6	3	3	4.4	800	kids, dogs
60 Carl Lake	7	4	5	9.8	1000	dogs
61 Duffy Lake	8	3	5	7	800	kids, dogs

MODERATE HIKES	Scenery	Solitude	Difficulty	Miles	Elev. Gain	Trail Use
1 Duckabush River Trail (last camp)	5	6	6	13.4	2800	
4 Goat Lake and Gobblers Knob	8	5	6	9	2850	dogs
7 Dumbbell and Sand Lakes Loop	6	5	6	11.3	1550	kids, dogs
10 Heart Lake	8	7	6	13.4	2400	dogs
11 Snowgrass Flat Loop	10	6	1	14.3	3000	
12 Dome Camp	9	6	3	14.2	1950	
14 Mount Margaret Backcountry Lakes	8	6	4	15.8	3100	
19 Foggy Flat	8	7	5	13.5	1300	dogs
20 High Camp and Killen Creek	9	6	4	8.4	2350	kids, dogs
21 Horseshoe Meadow	7	6	7	14	1400	dogs

	Scenery	Difficulty	Solitude	Miles	Elev. Gain	Trail Use
24 Lake Wapiki	7	6	6	9.6	2500	kids, dogs
25 Tillamook Head (north)	6	5	4	8.8	1200	
26 Cape Falcon to Short Sand Beach	7	5	4	11.8	1800	kids, dogs
29 Silver Star Mountain (east)	8	7	6	13.5	2600	dogs
31 Dublin Lake	7	7	7	13.8	4200	
32 Eagle Creek (upper camp)	9	6	2	16.8	1700	
33 Herman Creek (Cedar Swamp)	6	5	7	14.6	2850	kids, dogs
34 Warren Lake	6	6	6	6.8	2100	dogs
36 Cairn Basin	10	6	4	8.4	2000	dogs
38 Burnt Lake	7	5	3	5.4	1500	dogs
39 Cast Lake and Zigzag	7	6	6	10.6	2600	dogs
40 Paradise Park	7	5	3	10.1	2100	dogs
41 Elk Meadows Loop	7	7	5	13.7	2700	dogs
42 Salmon River Trail (full trail)	6	6	6	14.3	2700	dogs
44 Twin Lakes Loop	5	4	4	9	1500	kids, dogs
46 Lookout Mountain and Oval Lake	7	6	7	6.4	2050	dogs
49 High Lake	6	7	9	6.6	2300	
51 Serene Lake Loop	7	6	4	12	2050	kids
53 Twin Lakes	6	5	5	13.8	2950	dogs
54 Big Slide Lake	7	5	7	10.8	2325	dogs
56 Pyramid Lake	7	5	9	4.4	900	
58 Jefferson Park (west)	10	5	2	11.8	1900	
60 Carl Lake Loop	7	6	5	15.6	1900	dogs
61 Santiam Lake	8	4	5	9.6	1200	kids, dogs
63 Washington Ponds	5	5	7	12	1150	dogs
64 Cache Creek	7	5	9	5.5	900	dogs

DIFFICULT HIKES	Ratings (1–10)					
	Scenery	Difficulty	Solitude	Miles	Elev. Gain	Trail Use
2 Lake of the Angels	8	8	7	7.4	3400	
3 Upper Lena Lake	9	8	2	14.4	3900	
5 Indian Henrys Hunting Ground and Pyramid Park	9	9	5	18	4900	
6 Indian Bar and Cowlitz Park	9	8	2	15	4000	
9 Coyote Ridge Loop	8	9	8	25.4	4350	
13 Goat Mountain-Green River Loop	7	8	8	17.9	3700	
18 Dark Meadow via Jumbo Peak	8	8	8	14	3100	dogs
19 Avalanche Valley	10	10	5	24.4	4800	
21 Crystal Lake	7	8	7	20	1900	dogs
22 Sunrise Camp	9	8	5	8	2650	
31 Tanner Butte	7	9	7	22.4	4700	
33 Herman Creek Trail (Mud Lake)	6	8	7	19	3700	dogs
36 Elk Cove	10	7	4	13.6	2450	dogs
37 Yocum Ridge	9	9	5	18.6	4500	
49 High Lake	6	7	9	6.6	2300	
52 Peechuck Lookout	6	7	8	7.2	2200	
58 Jefferson Park (north)	10	7	2	13	2700	
59 Shale Lake Loop	8	7	3	17.7	3000	dogs
62 Three Fingered Jack Loop	9	8	5	20.5	3300	
63 George Lake	5	7	7	17.5	1600	dogs

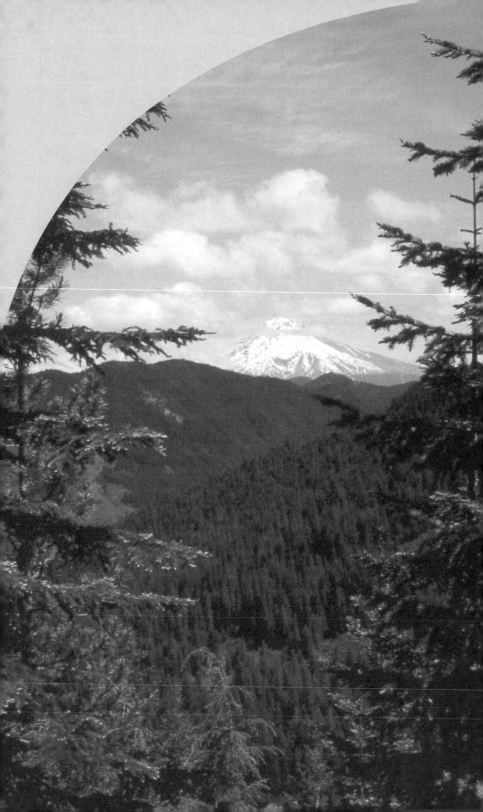

Introduction

As a child, I often dreamed of embarking on great backcountry adventures designed to test my outdoor skills in a remote wilderness setting. I would spend hours poring over maps of those increasingly rare but always enticing areas without any roads, planning out huge 100-mile-plus hikes to explore the imagined wonders within those boundaries. Invariably my visions included plenty of wildlife, outstanding scenery, and opportunities for both quiet introspection and grand adventure. In my youthful imagination these trips would last for several days or even weeks, a time span that, I thought, would allow me to fully immerse myself in the solitude and grandeur of the wilderness. In later years, I was lucky enough to take many such long adventures and even to write guidebooks describing some of my favorite long hikes.

I still take my share of long backpacking trips, but now that I am barreling headlong into middle age, nursing two long-suffering knees, and have a life that includes myriad other commitments, I am forced to put limits on my youthful ambitions. And I am not alone. Many of my fellow baby boomers no longer have the time, the energy, or the inclination to take the kinds of long backcountry adventures that they tackled in their youth. Instead, we seek out short mini-vacations (usually on weekends) to places where we can escape the rat race for a night or two, refresh our spirits, and then return to our busy lives with enough fond memories to sustain us until our next wilderness foray—always, so we fervently hope, not too far in the future.

Most of us are parents now, determined to drag our children away from the pervasive influence of video games and inane television fiction into the outdoors where they can experience the beautiful "real" world of nature. We do not, however, want that introduction to be so grueling that it will cause tired young legs to reject backpacking for the rest of their lives. Once again, short one-night hikes are what we seek, the kinds of relatively easy trips that get the kids excited about the outdoors, but don't cause too many sore muscles or painful blisters.

This book is designed with you in mind. The bookstore shelves are already filled with numerous dayhiking guides. I wrote one or two, and a few of the others are pretty good. But these volumes do not address the unique needs of the backpacker. Hikers looking for overnight adventures are forced to wade through dozens of trips that are unsuitable for backpacking in order to find the few that meet their needs. In addition, these guidebooks rarely provide the kind of information that is most useful to backpackers, such as specifically where to find the best campsites, the location of the nearest water source, or what overnight permits are required. All of these concerns are addressed here.

Since this book includes only the Portland area's best short backpacking options, it is not a comprehensive guide to *all* of the region's hundreds of overnight hiking possibilities. (See Appendix A, p. 212, for a more thorough listing.) It does, however, present a wide selection of outings, including a range of scenery and difficulty levels, so hikers of all abilities and interests will find plenty of trips to meet their needs.

Tips on Backpacking in the Pacific Northwest

Although this is more of a "where to go" book than a "how to" guide, it may be helpful, especially for those who are new to our area, to cover a few basic tips and ideas specific to backcountry travel in the Pacific Northwest.

GET THE RIGHT PERMITS: Most national forests in our region require that a Northwest Forest Pass be displayed in the windows of all vehicles parked within 0.25 mile of any major, developed trailhead. Isolated trailheads with minimal or no facilities are generally exempt. In 2008 daily permits were $5 and an annual pass was $30. The passes are available at ranger stations and at many local sporting goods stores, or they can be purchased online at www.naturenw.org/store-passes.htm.

CHECK THE SNOWPACK: The winter snowpack has a significant effect, not only on when a trail opens, but also on wildflower blooming times, peak stream flows, and how long seasonal water sources will be available. It is a good idea to check the snowpack on or about April 1 (the usual seasonal maximum), and make a note of how it compares to normal.

This information is available online at www.wa.nrcs.usda.gov/snow/ for Washington state and www.or.nrcs.usda.gov/snow/ for Oregon. If the snowpack is significantly above or below average, adjust the trip's seasonal recommendations accordingly.

WATCH OUT FOR LOGGING TRUCKS: When driving on forest roads in our area, keep a wary eye out for log trucks, especially on weekdays. These scary behemoths often barrel along with little regard for those annoying speed bumps known as passenger cars.

CHECK TRAIL CONDITIONS: The Northwest's frequently severe winter storms create annual problems for trail crews. Occasionally trails are washed out for years, but at a minimum, early-season hikers should expect to crawl over deadfall and search for routes around slides and flooded riverside trails. Depending on current funding and the trail's popularity, maintenance may not be completed until several weeks after a trail is snow-free and officially "open." Unfortunately, this means that trail maintenance is often done well after the optimal time to visit. On the positive side, trails are usually less crowded before the maintenance has been completed.

LEAF IT, DON'T LEAVE IT: For environmentally conscious backpackers, one good solution to the old problem of how to dispose of toilet paper is to find a natural alternative. Two excellent options are the large, soft leaves of thimbleberry at lower elevations, and the light-green lichen that hangs from trees at higher elevations. They're not exactly Charmin soft, but they get the job done.

WARN HUNTERS YOU'RE NOT A DEER: General deer-hunting season in Oregon and Washington runs from the second or third weekend of October to early November. For safety, anyone planning to travel on national or state forest land during these periods (particularly those doing any cross-country travel) should carry and wear a bright red or orange cap, vest, pack, or other conspicuous article of clothing. Hunting is not allowed in state or national parks, so this precaution does not apply to those areas.

YOU'RE NOT AN ELK, EITHER: Along the same line as the above, elk-hunting season is generally held in late October or early November. The exact season varies in different parts of each state.

BE CAREFUL WITH FUNGI: Mushrooms are a Northwest backcountry delicacy. Although our damp climate makes it possible to find mushrooms in any season, late August through November is usually best. Where and when the mushrooms can be found varies with elevation, precipitation, and other factors. Unfortunately, mushroom collecting has become a big and very competitive business in our region, and a few people have even been murdered in recent years in disputes over prize locations. Make sure any commercial collectors you meet are aware that you are only gathering a few mushrooms for personal use.

Also make absolutely sure that you know your fungi. There are several poisonous species of mushrooms in our forests, and every year people become ill or even die when they make a mistake in identification.

BRING THE BEATER: Car break-ins and vandalism, sadly, are regular occurrences at trailheads. This is especially true at popular trailheads and is a particular problem for backpackers who leave their vehicles unattended overnight. Thus, hikers need to take reasonable precautions. Do not encourage the criminals by providing unnecessary temptation. Preferably, leave the new car at home and drive to the trailhead in an older, beat-up vehicle. Even more importantly, leave nothing of value inside, especially in plain sight. My car has been broken into three times over the years. The last two times all the thieves managed to take home were some ratty old tennis shoes, to which they were welcome. If all trailhead vehicles held only items of similar value, the criminals would soon give up and seek out more lucrative targets.

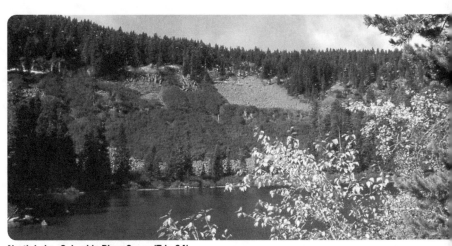

North Lake, Columbia River Gorge (Trip 34)

The 10 Essentials

Except when hiking on gentle trails in city parks, hikers should always carry a pack with certain essential items. The standard "10 Essentials" have evolved from a list of individual items to functional systems that will help to keep you alive and reasonably comfortable in emergency situations:

1. Navigation: topographic map and a compass or GPS device.

2. Sun protection: sunglasses and sunscreen, especially in the mountains.

3. Insulation: extra clothing that is both waterproof and warm.

4. Illumination: a flashlight or head-lamp.

5. First-aid supplies.

6. Fire: a candle or other firestarter and matches in a waterproof container.

7. Repair kit: particularly a knife for starting fires, first aid, and countless other uses.

8. Nutrition: enough extra food so you return with a little left over.

9. Hydration: extra water and a means to purify more on longer trips.

10. Emergency shelter: a tent, bivy sack, or emergency blanket.

I strongly advise adding a small plastic signaling whistle and a warm knit cap to this list.

Just carrying these items, however, does not make you "prepared." Unless you know things like how to apply basic first aid, how to build an emergency fire, and how to read a topographic map or use a compass, then carrying these items does you no good at all. These skills are all fairly simple to learn and at least one member of your group should be familiar with each of them.

More important to your safety and enjoyment than any piece of equipment or clothing is exercising common sense. When you are far from civilization, a simple injury can be life-threatening. Don't take unnecessary chances. Never, for example, jump onto slippery rocks or logs or crawl out onto dangerously steep slopes in the hope of getting a better view. Fortunately, the vast majority of wilderness injuries are easily avoidable.

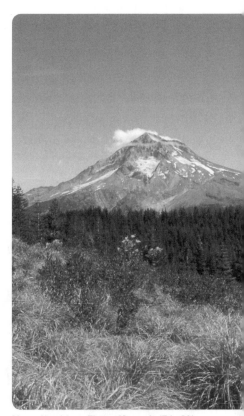

Mount Hood from Zigzag Mountain (Trip 39)

Advice for the First-Time Backpacker

This book is not a "how-to" manual for new backpackers. Entire books have been written on this subject, many of which are very good and well worth reading. (For recommendations, please turn to Appendix B, p. 222.) However, since every year thousands of people go backpacking for the first time, it is important to cover a few basics about making the transition from dayhiking to backpacking.

First and foremost, welcome! There is something enormously liberating about spending a night in the wilderness. Many of the Pacific Northwest's most spectacular attractions are beyond the reach of a comfortable dayhike, leaving them for the overnight hiker to enjoy.

Before joining the club of lucky souls out there sleeping under the stars, however, it is important that you go in with both eyes open (while you hike, that is, not while you sleep). Many people who regularly take dayhikes assume that backpacking is just dayhiking plus spending the night. Wrong! The two activities have some very important differences. For example, people often blithely assume that since they regularly go on dayhikes of 10 miles or more, they can cover the same distance when carrying overnight gear. This is a fundamental error because backpacking is an activity in which gravity displays its most sinister qualities. Believe me, your hips, shoulders, feet, knees, and probably a few body parts you had not even thought about in years will feel every extra ounce. And at least in compari-

son to dayhiking, backpacking requires carrying quite a few extra ounces.

Perhaps more importantly, backpacking calls for a different mental attitude. It is usually unwise, for example, to travel alone, at least on your first few trips. This advice applies even to people who regularly take solo dayhikes. Most people assume that this recommendation is for safety reasons, but while there is some safety in numbers, the main reason not to go backpacking alone is mental. Human beings are social animals. Most people enjoy backpacking (or any activity) much more if they have along at least one compatible companion with whom they can share the day's events and experiences. And having a hiking partner will make your journey more comfortable, because you can lighten your load by sharing the weight of community items such as a tent, a cook stove, and a water filter. If you haven't got the sales skills to talk reluctant friends or skeptical family members into coming along, consider joining a hiking club, where you will find plenty of people with similar outdoor interests. (See Appendix C, p. 224, for the names and addresses of some local organizations.)

Another thing that distinguishes backpacking from dayhiking is that backpackers need a different set of skills. They need to know how to hang their food to keep out bears and other critters. They need to know how to select an appropriate campsite—where breezes will keep the bugs away, where there aren't dangerous or unstable snags overhead, where the runoff from overnight rains won't create a lake beneath their tent, and a host of other variables. They need to know the optimal way to put things into their packs (where heavy items belong versus lighter ones) to carry a heavier load in

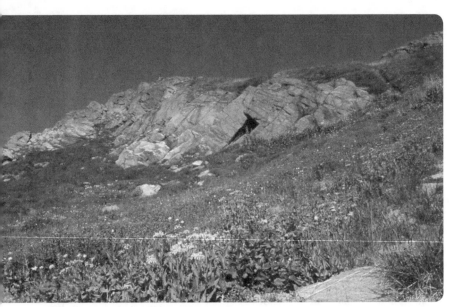

Flowers near Goat Lake, Goat Rocks Wilderness (Trip 11)

the most comfortable way possible. Although the list of skills is long, they are all interesting, relatively easy to learn, and well worth the time and effort to acquire. (Turn to the recommended reading section in Appendix B, p. 222, for a list of books that will help.)

Probably the most obvious difference between dayhiking and backpacking is the different equipment involved. Like dayhikers, all backpackers should carry the "10 Essentials" listed in the last section. But when you are spending the night, there are numerous other items you will need in order to remain safe and reasonably comfortable. A partial list of important items that every backpacker should carry but that dayhikers rarely need includes:

- A sleeping bag (preferably filled with synthetic material, since down doesn't work as well in our wet climate).

- A tent (with a rain fly, mosquito netting, and a waterproof bottom). Oh, and don't forget to run a test by putting the thing up in the backyard first, so you aren't trying to puzzle out how it works as a rainstorm starts in the backcountry and you discover you are three stakes short of accomplishing the task. (Don't ask me how I know this—just take my word for it.)

- A water filter or other water purification system.

- A lightweight sleeping pad for comfort and insulation against the cold ground.

- 50 feet of nylon cord to hang your food away from critters at night.

- Personal hygiene items.

- Insect repellent (especially in July and early August in the mountains).

- A lightweight backpacker's stove with fuel, cooking pots, and utensils if you want hot meals.

One final, important difference between dayhiking and backpacking, often overlooked, is that backpackers need to be much more careful to minimize their impact on the land. All hikers should do things like picking up litter, avoiding fragile vegetation, never cutting switchbacks, and leaving wildlife alone. For backpackers, however, there are some additional considerations. These are the some of the most important ones:

Since you'll probably be doing a lot of wandering around near camp, it is crucially important that you put your tent in a place that is either compacted from years of previous use or can easily take the impact without being damaged. A campsite on sand, rocks, or in a densely wooded area is best. Never camp on fragile meadow vegetation or immediately beside a lake or stream. If you see a campsite "growing" in an inappropriate location, be proactive: place a few limbs or rocks over the area to discourage further use, scatter "horse apples," and remove any fire-scarred rocks.

In a designated wilderness area, regulations generally require that you camp at least 100 feet from water. In places with long-established camps that are already heavily impacted, however, land managers usually prefer that you use the established site, even if it is technically too close to water, rather than trampling a new area.

Do not build campfires. Although fires were once a staple of camping and backpacking, today few areas can sustain the negative impact of fires. In many wilderness areas and national parks, fires are now officially prohib-ited, especially at higher elevations. For cooking, use a lightweight stove (they are more reliable, easier to use, and cleaner than fires). For warmth, try wearing a sweater or going for an evening stroll.

Finally, to have as little impact as possible, just throw water over yourself to remove the daily dirt and use biodegradable soap to clean your dishes well away from water sources. Backpackers should also leave at home any outdated attitudes about going out to "conquer" the wilderness.

Reintroducing Yourself to Backpacking

For many of you, it has probably been several years since you went on an overnight hike, so before hitting the trails, take the time for a quick refresher course. You may be surprised to discover how many things have changed. For example, although hiking still remains wonderfully free of restrictions, the wilderness is now increasingly regulated. Places that you previously visited on the spur of the moment may now require permits—to park at the trailhead, to spend the night, or even to hike the trail at all. On the positive side, equipment has changed radically in the last couple of decades, becoming much lighter and more efficient.

Step one for anyone contemplating a backpacking trip is to get into some kind of reasonable shape. Blisters while you hike and painfully sore muscles when you return are *not* badges of honor, they just *hurt*. Therefore, some simple, regular conditioning to get into reasonable aerobic shape, and strengthening key muscle groups (such as the calves, thighs, and shoulders) are crucial to having a good time.

Step two is to gather together all the gear you'll need. You remember, it's that pile of musty stuff in the basement that you haven't looked at in years, but which you haven't had the heart to give away since you always told yourself you'd be using it again. Pull it all out, clean things up, and check for and repair any damage, such as seams that have torn out, places where mice have chewed through the shoulder straps, and instances where the tent seams are no longer waterproof. Make sure things still fit properly (no offense, but that hip belt might need to be let out some). Finally, decide if you have everything you need and if what you have might be significantly improved. I am *not* suggesting that you spend a fortune on new gear. It is not necessary and, especially for the first few trips (until you decide you want to do this regularly), it is probably unwise. However, for a few items, especially the bulkiest and heaviest ones, you might consider upgrading.

With the extra load, backpacking usually requires better foot stability than dayhiking, so good boots are your first priority. For most trips, all you need are a sturdy pair of those new lightweight but still waterproof ones that are made partly of fabric and partly of leather. For longer and tougher outings, it is usually better to go with all-leather boots.

Once you have taken care of the footwear, it's time to turn to the rest of your body. Today's hiking clothes feature all kinds of terrific, hi-tech, lightweight fabrics that keep you warm on cold days and cooler on hot ones, that magically wick moisture away from your skin, resist getting smelly, and even have built-in bug repellent. Buying everything new would be prohibitively expensive, so focus first on investing in a pair of the new, decadently cushy, wool-blend socks and one of those nifty new undershirts that wick sweat away and are very comfortable. Once you are convinced of the benefits of the new clothing, turn to buying hiking shirts and pants that are made of a thin but remarkably tough nylon-blend fabric that stops the wind and dries extremely quickly.

As with clothing, almost every other piece of backpacking equipment has recently undergone design upgrades and changes in materials to make it noticeably lighter, stronger, and easier to use. Tents are now wonderfully light and easier to put up. Packs are better designed to fit your body. Sleeping pads are impressively cushy and comfortable. Sleeping bags fit better, last longer, and are much warmer. So if you are not satisfied with your current gear, head for the nearest sporting goods store, check out the product ratings in the hiking magazines, and do a little shopping. Your top priorities should be a comfortable pack and a lightweight tent.

Also, be sure to obtain a water filter or other modern method of water purification. Unfortunately, you can no longer drink untreated water out of most backcountry creeks and lakes, even if they look clear and pure. Nasty microorganisms live there and, believe me, you *really* don't want to ingest them.

In the late 1980s and early 1990s outdoor equipment manufacturers had one of those "Well, duh!" sort of epiphanies when they noticed, apparently for the first time, that men and women are different. This belated discovery has dramatically improved life for female backpackers, who were previously forced to use smaller versions of equipment designed for men. But today, women have a wide array of clothing, sleeping bags, packs, and accessories that are specifically designed to fit their body shape and unique needs. So if it has been several years since those of you proudly sporting two "X" chromosomes have been backpacking, you might want to look into upgrading your equipment. The added comfort and utility of the new female-oriented gear may make the cost worthwhile.

Introducing Your Kids to Backpacking

By the time I turned 12 years old, I had been going on dayhikes and family car-camping trips for well over half my life. Then, just as I was starting to get the hang of things, my father decided to up the ante and take me backpacking. Gallons of blood donated to thick clouds of mosquitoes turned that first trip into an unmitigated disaster, but youthful enthusiasm overrode good sense, and I was happily backpacking again the next weekend. Apparently, when you find the right mix of an active young mind and the wonders of nature, it is an irresistible (and a wonderful) combination.

Even though it requires considerably more work and planning, few things in life are more gratifying or enjoyable than taking a kid backpacking. One big reason for this is that children have the unique capacity to renew your appreciation of the outdoors. No mat-ter how commonplace and mundane things may be to you, *everything* is new and interesting to a child. The list of wonders includes all kinds of "little" things—mushrooms, old pine cones, tadpoles, fern fronds, discarded feathers—that adults no longer appreciate or even notice. In fact, it is downright humbling to see how much a child "notices," and the feeling is only slightly reduced by the realization that children possess a natural height advantage when it comes to seeing things that are close to the ground.

Although backpacking with a child may be fun for the adult, it is even better for the kid. Today, when American children spend, on average, more than *6 hours a day* (!) staring at some kind of electronic screen, and where even summer "camp" is more likely to be a computer camp than one where a kid can actually get outdoors, it is vital that we reintroduce our children to nature. A growing body of evidence indicates that regular contact with the outdoors is a natural antidote for attention deficit disorder, depression, and obesity, and is generally crucial for a child's overall mental and physical development. What better way to fill that need than to take them to a place where electronic screens simply aren't an option, and where they can explore a world filled with newts and flowers, pine cones and toads, and countless other real-world wonders?

To ensure that the backpacking experience is a great one (for both young and old), here are a few tips and guidelines to keep in mind:

- Despite everything you will read elsewhere (including in this introduction), when backpacking with young children, leave the teensy-ultralight-supposedly-for-two-people-but-only-if-they-are-on-their-honeymoon tent at home and pack along a nice roomy shelter.

- Don't forget that children, much more than adults, need a few comforts of home. Packing along that favorite blankie, stuffed animal, or bedtime storybook may be essential to everyone getting a good night's sleep.

- Remember that young bodies are less tolerant of weather extremes than older ones. Precautions such as protection from the sun, drinking plenty of water, and bundling up for the cold, for example, are all much more important for children than adults.

- Recognize that your kids, especially preteens, will get dirty—probably downright filthy, in fact. Live with it. Don't bother to scrub them clean every time you see them. A dirty kid usually means they are having fun.

- If your kids are too young to recognize natural dangers (poison oak, steep drop-offs, anthills, or the like) then you will need to physically block these off or post a watch among the adults.

- A little entertainment makes a big difference. In the evening, kids love the idea of having a headlamp (for some reason it's really cool), so bring along one for every member of the party. Bring simple games to keep everyone entertained in the evening. Playing cards, "pick-up sticks," and small board games all work well. Finally, don't forget to brush up on your storytelling. It is still the best way to spend an evening with kids in the outdoors.

- Don't forget to bring snacks. Lots of 'em.

- Be thoroughly familiar with child first aid, and recheck your first aid kit to ensure that it contains children's aspirin, lots of bandages (often great for psychological comfort even when the child isn't really hurt), and tweezers for removing splinters.

- Consider bringing along the child's best young human friend, or even their whole family. It may not fit with your idea of solitude in the wilderness, but kids usually love having a playmate while exploring the outdoors.

- How much leeway and independence you give your child depends on their age and responsibility level. You have to be able to trust that the youngster will follow instructions and not stray too far from camp when searching for huckleberries, chasing a squirrel, or some other equally distracting activity. To help combat this problem, all younger children should carry a whistle, preferably on a necklace, which they have been instructed to blow if (and only if) they become lost and need to be found.

Your choice of backpacking location is especially crucial when traveling with young hikers. Unlike adults, children are rarely impressed by great views and invariably complain about steep climbs. (To be fair, we adults often complain about steep climbs as well.) This book includes dozens of backpacking trips that are especially well suited to children. Identified both in the summary chart on pp. xii–xiii and by icons on the first page of the individual hike, these trips are relatively short, involve less elevation gain, and include plenty of the things that youngsters love—splashing creeks, wildlife, berries, lakes to explore, and the like.

An excellent time to schedule a backpacking trip with kids, especially into the Cascade Mountains, is late August. This is huckleberry season, when children (and adults) can stuff themselves with handfuls of the delicious berries. In fact, one measure of the success of a hike at this time of year is how purple one's fingers and tongue are by day's end. In addition, the mosquitoes are usually gone by this time, and the mountain lakes remain warm enough for a reasonably comfortable swim. Finally, your trip will take place just before kids go back to school, so they will have impressive stories to tell when their teacher asks the inevitable, "So, Suzy, what did *you* do this summer?"

For further information on backpacking with children, see the recommended reading in Appendix B, p. 222.

How to Use This Guide

The trips in this book are broken down by geographic region, starting from the southeastern Olympic Mountains in the north and working down to the Mt. Jefferson and Mt. Washington area in the south.

Each individual trip begins with a quick overview of the hike's vital statistics, including scenery, solitude, and difficulty ratings, as well as distance, elevation gain, managing agency, best time to visit, and more. This allows you to rapidly narrow your options based on your preferences, your abilities, and the time of year.

Just below the trip title are numerical **RATINGS** (1 to 10) of the three qualities that traditionally attract or deter hikers the most: the hike's scenery, its difficulty, and the degree of solitude you can expect.

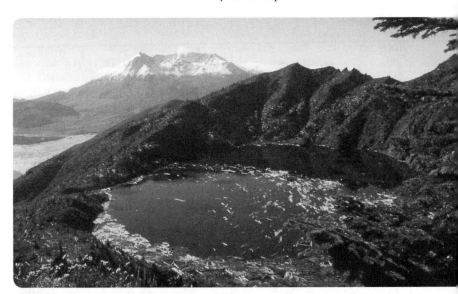

Mount Saint Helens and Saint Helens Lake (Trip 12)

Map Legend

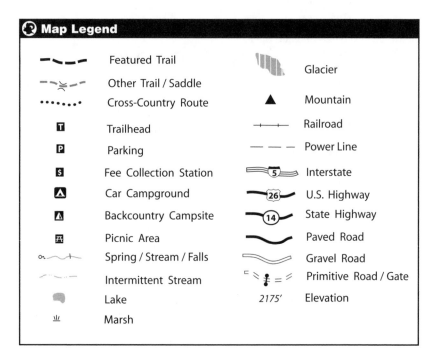

—∖—	Featured Trail		Glacier
—∖≋—	Other Trail / Saddle		
•••••••	Cross-Country Route	▲	Mountain
T	Trailhead	—+—+—	Railroad
P	Parking	— — —	Power Line
S	Fee Collection Station	⟨5⟩	Interstate
A	Car Campground	⟨26⟩	U.S. Highway
A	Backcountry Campsite	⟨14⟩	State Highway
A	Picnic Area		Paved Road
∿	Spring / Stream / Falls		Gravel Road
	Intermittent Stream	⊏∖↕=∠	Primitive Road / Gate
	Lake	*2175'*	Elevation
⋓	Marsh		

The **SCENERY** rating is my subjective opinion of the trip's overall scenic quality on a 1 (an eyesore) to 10 (absolutely gorgeous) scale. This rating reflects my personal biases in favor of photogenic views, clear streams, and wildflowers. If you prefer other qualities, then your own rating may be quite different. Also keep in mind that the rating is a relative one. All the trips in this book have beautiful scenery. Some are just better than others.

The **DIFFICULTY** rating is also subjective, and runs from 1 (barely leave the La-Z-Boy) to 10 (the Ironman Triathlon). Since most out-of-shape Americans would find even the easiest backpacking trip to be very strenuous, this rating is relative only to other trips.

Since **SOLITUDE** is one of the things backpackers are seeking, it helps to know roughly how much company you can expect. This rating is also on a 1 (bring stilts to see over the crowds) to 10 (just you and the marmots) scale. Of course, even on a "10" hike, it is possible that you could unexpectedly run into a pack of unruly Cub Scouts, but generally this rating is pretty accurate.

The next two lines list total **ROUND-TRIP DISTANCE** and **ELEVATION GAIN** for that trip. For many hikers, the difficulty of a trip is determined more by how far up they go than the mileage they cover, so pay especially close attention to the second number, which includes the total of all ups and down, not merely the net change in elevation.

OPTIONAL MAP: Every trip includes a map that is as up-to-date and as accurate as possible. Many hikers, however, will also want to carry a topographic map. This entry identifies the best available map(s) for the described trip.

Next you will find two seasonal entries. The **USUALLY OPEN** line tells you when a trip is typically snow-free enough for hiking (which can vary considerably from year to year). The second entry lists the particular **BEST TIME(S)** of year when the trip is at its very best (when the flowers peak, or the huckleberries are ripe, or the mosquitoes have died down, etc.).

AGENCY: This is the local land agency responsible for the area described in the hike. (See Appendix D, p. 225, for contact information.)

PERMIT: This section tells you if a permit is currently required to enter or camp in the area and how to obtain one. It notes the few instances when the permits are not free or where advanced reservations are required, and provides the necessary details. When a Northwest Forest Pass is required to park at the trailhead, this is also indicated.

ICONS AND TRAIL USES: If they're appropriate for children or dogs, the trips in this book will be labeled with an icon.

 This hike is good for children.

 Pets are allowed and the trail is both safe and suitable for dogs.

HIGHLIGHTS: This section summarizes the most interesting features of a particular trip, letting you quickly assess whether it's what you're looking for.

GETTING THERE: This section provides driving directions to the trailhead from Portland.

HIKING IT: In this section, your hiking route is described in detail beginning at the trailhead and through each trail junction you'll encounter.

Safety Notice

While backpacking is not an inherently dangerous sport, there are certain risks you take any time you venture away from the comforts of civilization. The trips in this book go through remote wilderness terrain. In an emergency, medical supplies and facilities will not be immediately available. The fact that a hike is described in this book does not mean that it will be safe for you. Hikers must be properly equipped and in adequate physical condition to handle a given trail. Because trail conditions, weather, and hikers' abilities all vary considerably, the author and the publisher cannot assume responsibility for anyone's safety. Use plenty of common sense and a realistic appraisal of your abilities, and you will be able to enjoy these trips safely.

References to "water" in the text attest only to its availability, not its purity. All backcountry water should be treated before you drink it.

Southeastern Olympic Mountains

The Olympic Mountains fill the center of the Olympic Peninsula, a wild extension of land in western Washington that is separated from the rest of our region by Puget Sound and its numerous tidal arms. This was one of the last areas in the Lower 48 to be explored, and to this day much of the peninsula remains wonderfully wild, thanks largely to the protection provided by Olympic National Park. Although relatively low in elevation (the highest peaks are only around 7000 feet), the mountains are remarkably "tall," because they begin practically at sea level. They are also exceptionally rugged, having been eroded into sharp ridges and deep valleys by ancient glaciers and the enormous quantities of rain that continue to fall today. Only a small portion of the far southeastern edge of this range is close enough to Portland to make a reasonable weekend destination, but that sampling is well worthwhile and, with the exception of lush rain forests, it includes all of the attributes found elsewhere in these mountains: plenty of wildflowers, abundant wildlife, lovely streams and lakes, and terrific mountain scenery.

1 Duckabush River Trail

RATINGS	Scenery **5** Difficulty **2 to 6** Solitude **6**
ROUND-TRIP DISTANCE	4.4 miles to first camp; 13.4 miles to park boundary
ELEVATION GAIN	900 feet to first camp; 2800 feet to park boundary
OPTIONAL MAP	*Green Trails: The Brothers*
USUALLY OPEN	April to November
BEST TIMES	Late April to June / October
AGENCY	Hood Canal Ranger District (Olympic National Forest)
PERMIT	Park service permit required if you camp beyond 6.7 miles from the trailhead. Permits cost $5 to register your group, plus $2 per person per night. Contact the park's wilderness information center for permits. Northwest Forest Pass required.

Highlights

Although it features some exceptionally nice views along the way, the Duckabush River Trail is primarily a forest hike that follows one of the largest and most important rivers flowing out of the eastern Olympic Mountains. Since the trail is open for most of the year, this is a particularly good choice for a spring or fall adventure, when the higher mountains are still encased in snow.

Getting There

Drive 110 miles north of Portland on Interstate 5 to Olympia and take Exit 104 for U.S. Highway 101. After 6 miles, exit to the right, staying on Highway 101, and then drive 50 miles to a junction with paved Duckabush River Road near Milepost 310. Turn left (west), drive 6.1 miles on pavement then good gravel to a junction, bear right, and reach the road-end trailhead after another 0.2 mile.

Hiking It

The gravel-strewn trail begins on a hillside well away from the river as it makes a gentle climb through a forest of Douglas firs and western hemlocks. After gaining 450 feet in 1.2 miles, the trail reaches the relatively unimpres-

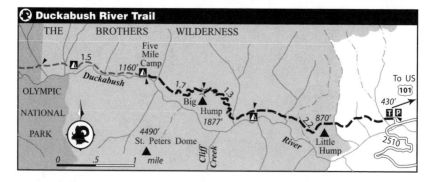

Duckabush River Trail

THE   BROTHERS   WILDERNESS

OLYMPIC
NATIONAL
PARK

Five
Mile
Camp

1.5   1160'

Duckabush

1.7

Big
Hump
1877'

4490'
St. Peters Dome

1.3

870'

River

2.2

Little
Hump

To US
101

430'

2510

0   .5   1   mile

sive top of a rocky spur called Little Hump. From here you descend all the way to the river and walk across lush river-level flats filled with old stumps (testament to the logging that once occurred here) and a vigorous second-growth forest of Douglas firs, maples, and countless thousands of ferns. At 2.2 miles is an excellent campsite beside the clear Duckabush River. If you are backpacking with children, this is a good place to spend the night.

Beyond the first camp you face the trip's biggest obstacle, a 1000-foot climb over the top of Big Hump. This rocky mass, which was left behind by ancient glaciers, requires two dozen short, fairly steep, and rather tiring switchbacks to conquer. Fortunately, partway up is a perfect rest stop at a fine overlook with a superb view of the forested Duckabush Valley. Across the valley to the south rises prominent St. Peters Dome, whose towering sheer sides make it look as if it were transplanted from California's Yosemite Valley. Beyond this viewpoint more uphill takes you past a nice but not as impressive viewpoint before you come to the indistinct top of Big Hump in viewless forest.

It is nearly all downhill from here as switchbacks descend 700 feet to the cascading Duckabush River just above where the water cuts a gorge around Big Hump. Not far upstream is Five Mile Camp (actually at 5.2 miles, but close enough), a comfortable site with room for a few tents. Beyond here the trail stays in valley forests, making many small ups and downs but never straying too far from the water. There are several possible campsites along the way, but if you go beyond 6.7 miles, where the trail enters the national park, you will need a Park Service permit to spend the night. The park also prohibits firearms and pets. Hardy hikers can continue their wilderness adventure, reaching lovely Ten Mile Camp at (you guessed it) a little over 10 miles, and eventually climbing to the gorgeous high meadows and lakes around Marmot Lake and O'Neil Pass. Both of these destinations are more than 20 miles into the heart of the glorious Olympic backcountry.

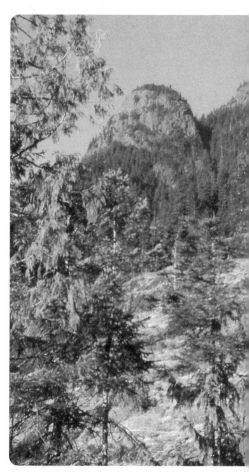

St. Peters Dome from Duckabush River Trail, Olympic National Forest

2 | Lake of the Angels

RATINGS	Scenery **8** Difficulty **8** Solitude **7**
ROUND-TRIP DISTANCE	7.4 miles
ELEVATION GAIN	3400 feet
OPTIONAL MAPS	*Green Trails: The Brothers, Mount Steel*
USUALLY OPEN	Mid-July to October
BEST TIMES	Mid-July to October
AGENCY	Hood Canal Ranger District (Olympic National Forest) and Olympic National Park
PERMIT	Park Service permit required for camping at the lake. Permits cost $5 to register your group, plus $2 per person per night. Contact the park's wilderness information center for permits.

Highlights

Although relatively short, this is a steep and challenging hike that takes you to a wonderfully scenic little alpine lake high in the Olympic Mountains. In addition to being a great destination in itself, the lake is a fine place to set up a base camp for explorations of the surrounding mountains. Due to the steepness and exposure of this route, those who are afraid of heights should not attempt this hike. Boots with good traction are a must, especially if conditions are wet.

Getting There

Drive 110 miles north of Portland on Interstate 5 to Olympia and take Exit 104 for U.S. Highway 101. After 6 miles you exit to the right, staying on Highway 101, and then drive 43.8 miles to a junction with paved Hamma Hamma River Road near Milepost 318. Turn left (west), drive 6.5 miles to a T junction, turn right, and then go 5.7 miles first on pavement then good gravel to the signed Putvin Trailhead immediately after a bridge over Boulder Creek.

Hiking It

The trail begins as a well-maintained path that climbs moderately steeply through a second-growth forest of western hemlocks and western red cedars. Salal, vine maple, sword fern, and Oregon grape are abundant beneath the forest canopy. On your right, generally unseen Boulder Creek cascades along in a nearly continuous waterfall. At 0.3 mile you pass the signed but easy-to-miss gravesite of Carl Putvin, who, the sign informs you, was a "pioneer, trapper, and explorer" who lived from 1892 to 1913. About 0.2 mile above this point, the trail climbs steeply around some huge moss-covered boulders before cutting to the left away from the creek and traveling at a gentler grade across a hillside. A few partial breaks in the forest here reveal tantalizing glimpses of rugged Mt. Pershing to the south.

At 1 mile you cross a pair of rocky gullies where the trail is prone to washouts. In another 0.3 mile you meet a long-abandoned road. Turn left (slightly downhill), and walk 25 yards to the resumption of the trail.

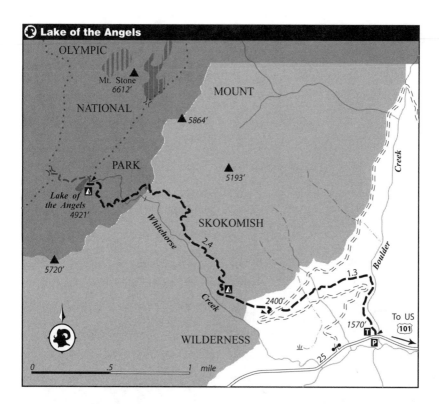

The now almost continuously steep trail makes a few short switchbacks, and then traverses to a sign indicating your entry into the Mount Skokomish Wilderness. Shortly beyond this sign, at 1.7 miles, and just before you come to (but do not cross) tumbling White-horse Creek, is a mediocre campsite on the right. From here more very steep uphill in short switchbacks leads to a relatively open avalanche chute at 2.3 miles that is choked with bracken fern, beargrass, and pearly everlasting.

Just 0.2 mile after the avalanche chute you reach a gently sloping basin filled with an impenetrable tangle of slide alder. Directly ahead of you, at the northwest end of this basin, is a steep headwall where waterfalls cascade down from above. Lake of the Angels

sits at the top of this imposing head-wall. The rough trail climbs around the right side of the basin and then charges very steeply uphill, often over exposed rocks. In a couple of places you will need to grab onto rocks and roots to help pull yourself up.

Near the top of the headwall, the terrain opens up, becomes less steep, and features lots of huckleberries and good views. The trail's last 0.5 mile goes up and down, crossing a marshy meadow and several small creeks, and passing a shallow pond before depositing you on the northeast shore of Lake of the Angels. This very scenic, teardrop-shaped lake is surrounded by rocky areas, meadows, and high-elevation conifers such as subalpine firs, Alaska yellow cedars, and mountain

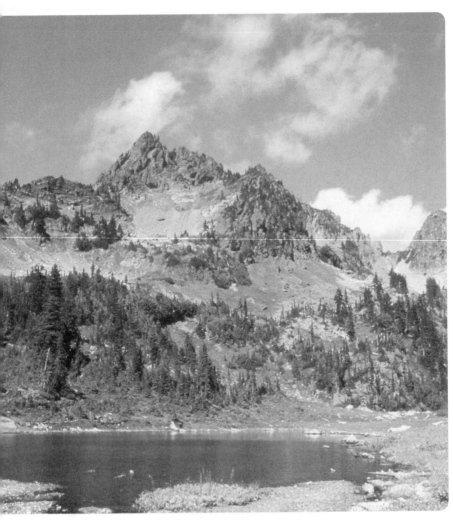

Mount Stone over Lake of the Angels, Olympic National Park

hemlocks. As always, never camp in the fragile meadows near the lake, but instead seek out places with harder surfaces away from the shore. The best views are from the south shore up to rugged Mt. Stone.

Adventurous hikers can use the lake as a base camp for some fine explorations. Top goals include the views from atop the ridge to the west (accessible by an easy but unsigned boot path), the Stone Ponds (reached by a tough scramble through an obvious notch in the southeast shoulder of Mt. Stone), and the top of a snow-filled gully high on the shoulder of Mt. Skokomish to the southwest.

3 | Lena Lakes

RATINGS	Scenery **9** Difficulty **4 to 8** Solitude **2**
ROUND-TRIP DISTANCE	6.2 miles to Lena Lake; 14.4 miles to Upper Lena Lake
ELEVATION GAIN	1350 feet to Lena Lake; 3900 feet to Upper Lena Lake
OPTIONAL MAP	*Green Trails: The Brothers*
USUALLY OPEN	April to November for Lena Lake; July to October for Upper Lena Lake
BEST TIMES	Any time it's open
AGENCY	Hood Canal Ranger District (Olympic National Forest) and Olympic National Park
PERMIT	Park Service permit required for camping at Upper Lena Lake. Permits cost $5 to register your group, plus $2 per person per night. Contact the park's wilderness information center for permits. Northwest Forest Pass required.

to lower
lake

Highlights

This trip gives you a choice. For an easier hike, follow the very popular trail to attractive Lena Lake, a lower-elevation destination that is open for most of the year. For more dramatic scenery, continue on a rougher trail that takes you into the high country around spectacular Upper Lena Lake, one of the most beautiful lakes in the Olympic Mountains. Hikers with children younger than teenagers should stop at Lena Lake.

Getting There

Drive 110 miles north of Portland on Interstate 5 to Olympia and take Exit 104 for U.S. Highway 101. After 6 miles you exit to the right, staying on Highway 101, and then drive 43.8 miles to a junction with paved Hamma Hamma River Road near Milepost 318. Turn left (west), drive 6.5 miles to a T junction, turn right, and then go another 1.3 miles to the well-signed Lena Lake Trailhead.

Hiking It

The wide, heavily traveled, and gently graded trail soon leaves the river bottom environment dominated by moss-draped bigleaf maples and gradually ascends a tangled forest of second-growth Douglas firs, western red cedars, and western hemlocks. The first 1.5 miles climb 14 switchbacks on a forested hillside before entering the lush canyon of loudly cascading Lena Creek. At 1.9 miles the trail crosses the creek on an unnecessarily large wooden bridge at a point where the stream flows underground and the creekbed is usually dry.

After the crossing, three more gentle switchbacks and a lengthy traverse lead to the south end of Lena Lake. Unfortunately, it is initially hard to get a good view of this large, deep, green-tinged lake, since the trail stays on the heavily forested hillside well above the western shore. At 3 miles the trail splits. The trail to the right leads past a fine rocky viewpoint above Lena Lake before passing numerous excellent campsites on the lake's northwest and north shores. This is where hikers with children or those looking for a relatively easy hike should call it a night. Fires are allowed only in established campsites with metal fire rings.

To reach Upper Lena Lake, take the left fork (uphill) at the trail split and follow a narrower trail that winds mostly uphill into the canyon of Lena Creek. After 0.4 mile go straight at the unsigned junction with a trail turning sharply right back toward Lena Lake. Your trail, which is rough in a few places but easy to follow, continues up the canyon, and at 4.2 miles passes a sign marking your entry into Olympic National Park. Pets and weapons are prohibited beyond this point.

At 5 miles you cross a side creek on a convenient log, after which the trail gets steeper, with more roots, rocks, and mud. Even with these obstacles, however, the route remains obvious and is not overly difficult. Numerous short, steep switchbacks now guide you into the high country, where forest openings provide enticing views to the east down the canyon of Lena Creek and up to a rugged ridge on the southwest shoulder of The Brothers. The trail makes a bridgeless crossing of Lena Creek at 6.3 miles just below a sliding waterfall, and then ascends several more short switchbacks to an open slope with fine views to the south of pyramid-shaped Mt. Bretherton. Finally, at 7.2 miles, you reach a junction just above the northeast shore of Upper Lena Lake.

This gorgeous lake, which sits in the basin between Mt. Lena to the north and Mt. Bretherton to the

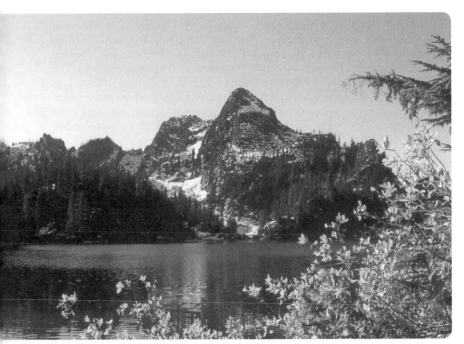

Mount Bretherton over Upper Lena Lake, Olympic National Park

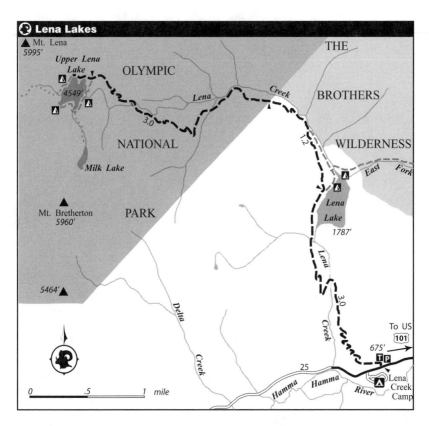

south, is rimmed with forests of mountain hemlock and Alaska yellow cedar and open areas featuring an abundance of pink heather. Fires are not allowed at the lake, and hikers are required to camp in designated sites on the lake's northwest, southeast, east, and southwest shores. Toilets and bear wires for hanging food are provided for your convenience.

The lake is ideal for setting up camp and doing some exploring. A top goal is the rough boot path that goes west over a low pass before continuing to Scout Lake (no camping allowed) and the tiny but dramatically scenic Stone Ponds. You can also follow a scramble route to the top of Mt. Lena or go south into the narrow basin holding Milk Lake.

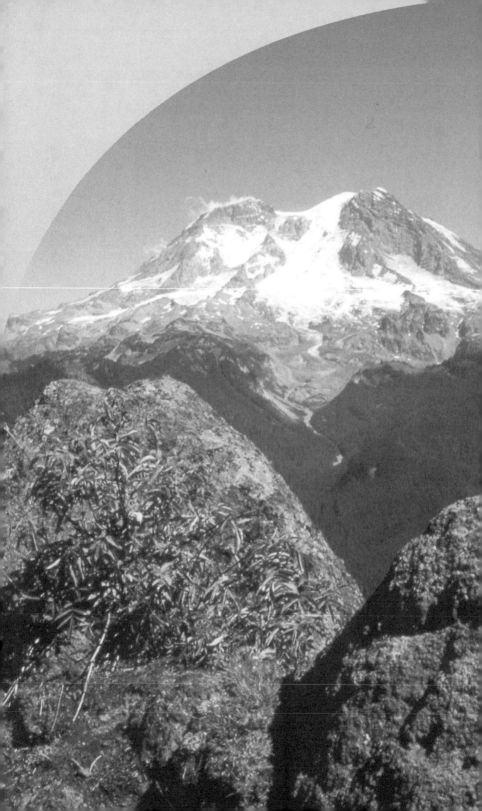

Southern Mount Rainier and the Goat Rocks

The undisputed king of the Cascade Mountains, Mt. Rainier rises 14,410 feet into the Pacific Northwest sky and is visible for hundreds of miles in every direction. The national park that surrounds the mountain is a national treasure and is much beloved, not only by locals but by admiring tourists from around the world. Only the southern part of the mountain is close enough for a reasonable weekend trip from Portland, but that includes some of the park's best scenery, including amazingly abundant wildflowers, enormous glaciers, stunning mountain views, plenty of wildlife, dozens of waterfalls—the list of wonders is almost endless.

Not far to the southeast of Mt. Rainier is a less famous, but no less worthy, mountain treasure: the Goat Rocks, the ruggedly scenic remains of an eroded volcano. The trails in both areas are justifiably popular, but with reservations in the national park and careful planning in the Goat Rocks Wilderness, it is possible to enjoy a welcome degree of solitude in your backcountry adventures. Even without solitude, the outstanding mountain scenery in both areas will delight you and keep you coming back time and again.

4 Goat Lake and Gobblers Knob

RATINGS	Scenery **8** Difficulty **5** Solitude **6**
ROUND-TRIP DISTANCE	6.8 miles to Goat Lake; 9 miles to Gobblers Knob
ELEVATION GAIN	1650 feet to Goat Lake; 2850 feet to Gobblers Knob
OPTIONAL MAP	*Green Trails: Mount Rainier West*
USUALLY OPEN	Mid-July to October
BEST TIMES	Mid-July to October
AGENCY	Cowlitz Valley Ranger District (Gifford Pinchot National Forest) and Mount Rainier National Park
PERMIT	None

Highlights

The tiny Glacier View Wilderness, which borders the west side of Mount Rainier National Park, includes similar scenery to the park, but avoids that more famous preserve's traffic jams and crowds. Long-distance hiking is limited by the small size of the wilderness, so most people who come here are day-hikers. The area is large enough, however, for a wonderful one-night outing to quiet Goat Lake with access to a spectacular view of Mt. Rainier from Gobblers Knob.

Getting There

Leave Interstate 5 north of Vancouver at Exit 68 and travel 31 miles east on U.S. Highway 12 to a junction at the town of Morton. Turn left on State Highway 7 and drive 17 miles to a junction with Highway 706. Turn right (east), proceed 11.1 miles to an unsigned junction near Milepost 11, and then turn left on gravel Forest Road 59. After climbing for 4.3 miles, turn sharply right on Road 5920 and slowly drive 1.6 miles on this rough and rocky road to the road-end trailhead.

Hiking It

The Lake Christine Trail starts in an ancient clear-cut now populated with 40-foot-tall Douglas firs and Pacific silver firs growing above a tangled mix of thimbleberry bushes, Sitka alders, fireweed, pearly everlastings, and various other shrubs, wildflowers, and grasses. The rocky path climbs very steeply for 0.1 mile, and then becomes more moderate when it enters uncut forest. In one switchback the intermittently steep path ascends through forest, and then across a hillside choked with elderberries, bluebells, salmonberries, cow parsnips, devils clubs, stinging nettles, and various other moisture-loving flowers and shrubs. At the top of the ascent, 0.8 mile from the trailhead, you arrive at the forested bowl holding tiny and rather shallow Lake Christine. Backed by a rugged but unnamed ridge to the east, this pretty little lake has nice views and features plenty of heather and other colorful wildflowers around its shore.

The trail circles to the right around the lake's south and east shores before

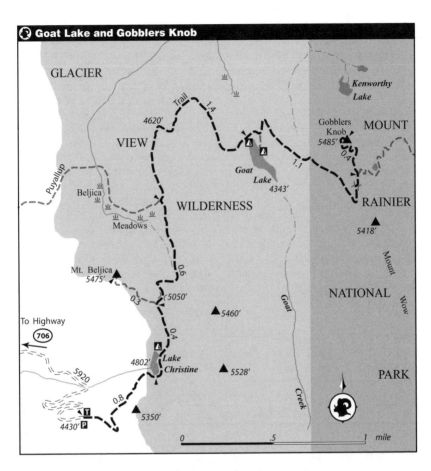

Goat Lake and Gobblers Knob

GLACIER

Kenworthy Lake

4620'

Gobblers Knob 5485'   MOUNT

VIEW

Trail 1.4

Goat Lake 4343'

1.1

Puyallup

Beljica

Meadows

WILDERNESS   RAINIER

5418'

Mt. Beljica 5475'

0.6

0.3 5050'

5460'

To Highway 706

NATIONAL

Goat

Mount Wow

0.4

4802' Lake Christine

5528'

PARK

5920

0.8

4430'

5350'

Creek

0   .5   1 mile

reaching a pair of nice campsites just after a log bridge over the tiny inlet creek. From here the path pulls away from the lake and slowly climbs a meadowy ravine that is alive with midsummer wildflowers such as bistort, aster, wild carrot, Sitka valerian, arnica, groundsel, and pink heather. At 1.2 miles is a signed junction with a spur trail to the viewpoint atop Mt. Beljica. This makes a good side trip, although better views will come later in the hike.

Go right at the junction, pass through a forested saddle, and then make a winding descent to a junction with Puyallup Trail at 1.8 miles. Turn right on this gently rolling trail as it rounds the north end of a ridge and then gradually descends to a nice campsite at the northern tip of Goat Lake at 3 miles. Although not spectacularly scenic, this long and narrow lake is very lovely, surrounded by stately forest with a narrow strip of grasses and flowers along the shore. The only views are of the long ridge of Mt. Wow rising to the southeast. For a larger and better campsite, continue on the trail that goes east and a bit uphill from Goat Lake for 0.1 mile, and then turn right on an obvious path that goes downhill for about 150 yards to an attractive camp on the east shore of Goat Lake.

So far the scenery on this hike has been pleasant, but not particularly dramatic. For a big scenic payoff, set up camp at Goat Lake and spend the afternoon on a side trip to the top of Gobblers Knob. From the junction with the access trail to the camp on Goat Lake's east shore, take the main trail, which steadily ascends a forested hillside and enters Mount Rainier National Park after about 0.5 mile. Firearms, livestock, and pets are prohibited beyond this point. The trail then continues uphill, now mostly over open slopes, to a minor saddle at the top of a ridge. Just 100 yards down the other side of the ridge is a junction. Veer left (uphill) on the Gobblers Knob Trail and in 0.4 mile ascend 10 well-graded switchbacks to the staffed lookout building perched atop the rocky summit.

The views of the route of this hike to the west are superb, but you probably won't notice them since your attention will be drawn to the east and the breathtaking view of the towering mass of nearby Mt. Rainier. Huge Tahoma Glacier tumbles down in an awesome display of white, while below that is a mantle of alpine meadows, rocky ridges, and forested valleys. This is one of the best views of the mountain anywhere. After plenty of time spent staring in awe, return the way you came.

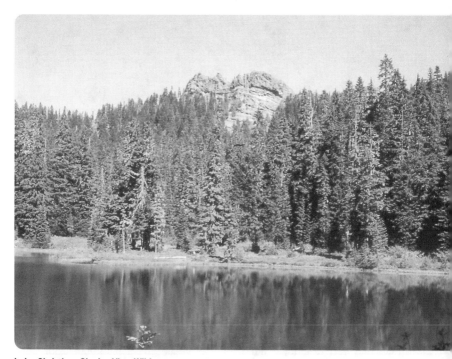

Lake Christine, Glacier View Wilderness

5 Indian Henrys Hunting Ground and Pyramid Park

RATINGS	Scenery **9** Difficulty **9** Solitude **5**
ROUND-TRIP DISTANCE	18 miles
ELEVATION GAIN	4900 feet
OPTIONAL MAP	*Green Trails: Mount Rainier West*
USUALLY OPEN	Late July to October
BEST TIMES	Late July to October
AGENCY	Mount Rainier National Park
PERMIT	Required. Reservations are strongly advised. All cars must also display an entry permit for the national park.
INFORMATION RESERVATION	Mount Rainier National Park sets aside only 40 percent of its available backcountry permits on a first-come, first-served basis. The remaining permits are given to hikers who made advance reservations. Since obtaining a permit for popular areas, especially on summer weekends, is extremely difficult, it is highly recommended that you reserve a permit in advance. Reservations are accepted starting on March 15 by mail, fax, or in person at the Longmire Wilderness Information Center. You cannot make a reservation over the phone. The cost is $20 per group and is nonrefundable. To obtain a reservation form and for further information, go to www.nps.gov/mora/planyourvisit/wilderness-reservation-information.htm.

Highlights

Indian Henrys Hunting Ground is one of the most famous backcountry beauty spots in Mount Rainier National Park. This glorious meadow, with its bonanza of wildflowers, scenic ponds, and drop-dead-gorgeous views of Mt. Rainier certainly deserves the fame, but all that popularity has forced the park to protect this fragile area by closing the meadow to camping. Most hikers approach Indian Henrys along the Wonderland Trail from Longmire and spend the night at crowded Devils Dream Camp, a little over 1 mile to the south. But for adventuresome hikers who are willing to do some moderate cross-country hiking, there is a better and less crowded option. By hiking into Indian Henrys Hunting Ground on the little-used Kautz Creek Trail and continuing up to spectacular but off-trail Pyramid Park, you can avoid the crowds and spend the night at an amazingly beautiful alpine retreat with a dramatic up-close look at the rugged west face of Mt. Rainier.

Getting There

Leave Interstate 5 north of Vancouver at Exit 68 and travel 31 miles east on U.S. Highway 12 to a junction at the town of Morton. Turn left on State Highway 7 and drive 17 miles to a

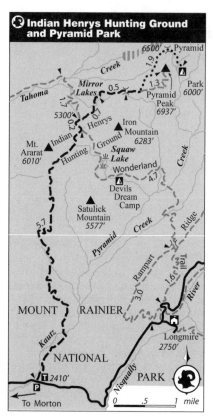

Indian Henrys Hunting Ground and Pyramid Park

junction with Highway 706. Turn right (east), enter Mount Rainier National Park after 14 miles, and continue another 3.4 miles to the Kautz Creek Trailhead. The parking lot is on the right. To obtain a permit (or to pick up your *reserved* permit) you will need to continue driving another 3 miles to Longmire and stop in at the wilderness information center.

Hiking It

The trail starts next to a small sign on the north side of the highway across from the parking lot. Initially the path takes you over the remains of a massive debris and mud flow that devas-

tated this valley in October 1947. The flow was triggered by heavy rains, which caused a partial collapse of the Kautz Glacier. Landslide events like this are fairly common on Mt. Rainier, although they are usually smaller in size. As recently as the fall of 2006, over 18 inches of rain fell in one day, which caused such extensive damage many park roads and trails had to be closed for the entire summer of 2007. For the next few years you should expect to encounter damage along many of the park's trails, so be sure to check on conditions before hiking this route. On the remains of the 1947 slide, small trees now crowd the area, mostly western hemlocks and western red cedars, but in more open and sunny areas deciduous trees, especially red alders, predominate. The dense undergrowth is mostly composed of salal, along with various ferns and mosses.

Initially the trail is very gentle, wide, and strewn with gravel to accommodate tourists interested in exploring the geology of the mudflow. At 1 mile, however, the trail crosses silty Kautz Creek on a seasonally-installed log bridge and becomes a wilderness trail. The much narrower path now enters an old-growth forest unaffected by the 1947 mudflow and begins a long, persistent, and at times moderately steep climb. The way is viewless but shady and pleasant throughout. Numerous short switchbacks help keep the climb from becoming overly steep. You cross a trickling creek at about 3 miles (the first reliable source of clear water), then climb some more in a series of short, steep switchbacks. Still not done with the uphill, you ascend at a gentler grade on a wide ridge and slowly enter more open high-elevation terrain. Mt. Rainier is frequently in view, while

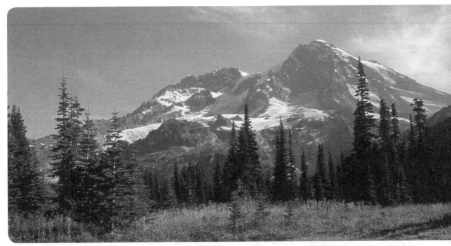

Mount Rainier over Indian Henrys Hunting Ground, Mount Rainier National Forest

closer at hand are rocky buttes and increasing numbers of heather, huck-leberries, and various wildflowers. A final short, steep uphill leads to a high point on the southeast shoulder of Mt. Ararat (a name that significantly over-states the size of this small butte), and then you descend about 150 feet to a junction at 5.7 miles with the Wonderland Trail.

You are now smack in the middle of Indian Henrys Hunting Ground, a spectacular mountain meadow with acres of colorful wildflowers, several tiny ponds, a small ranger cabin, and some of the most photogenic views of Mt. Rainier in the entire park. You turn left at the junction, almost immediately pass a spur trail to the ranger cabin, and 0.2 mile later come to a junction with the Mirror Lakes Trail. Turn right and gradually ascend 0.7 mile in rolling, wildflower-filled meadows to shallow Mirror Lake. Asahel Curtis made this view famous when he painted it for a postage stamp commemorating the national park in 1934. The scene is just as impressive today.

The trail rounds the right side of the tiny lake, and then goes 100 yards to a sign saying END OF MAINTAINED TRAIL. Despite its now unofficial status, the trail remains very good and easy to follow as it climbs for 0.4 mile, and then descends a bit to a meadow-filled saddle with a great view of aptly-named Pyramid Peak to the northeast. From here the trail continues to the top of Pyramid Peak, where you'll enjoy an absolutely out-of-this-world view of nearby Mt. Rainier.

Since there is nowhere to camp on Pyramid Peak, backpackers should go instead to Pyramid Park, a more dif-ficult-to-reach but equally spectacular destination. To reach it, follow the trail toward Pyramid Peak from the meadowy saddle for about 0.3 mile, and then go cross-country to the left, angling moderately steeply uphill to a rocky, above-timberline ledge on the northeast side of Pyramid Peak. Follow this rugged ledge for about 0.8 mile to a high, often windy saddle north of the peak, where you will enjoy up-close-and-personal views of Mt. Rainier that are so incredible the word "great" just doesn't do them justice.

From this rocky saddle you scramble steeply downhill, going southeast across boulder fields, meadows, and scree slopes to the rolling meadowlands, springs, and tree islands of Pyramid Park. Tall but unnamed waterfalls drop into and off the edge of this alpine parkland, while the banks of the gently meandering creeks that cross the flats are choked with yellow monkeyflowers, western anemones, grass-of-Parnassus, and other wildflowers. There are also great views to the west of Pyramid Peak and northeast to Mt. Rainier, which has a rather lopsided appearance from this angle. More distant views extend to the south and southeast of the Tatoosh Range, Mt. Adams, the Goat Rocks, and Mt. St. Helens. You can camp almost anywhere in this parkland, although, as always, you should select a rocky or sandy area that is well away from the delicate alpine wildflowers and grasses. If you schedule more than one night here, you can visit all of the waterfalls and enjoy the excellent scenery.

6 Indian Bar and Cowlitz Park

RATINGS	Scenery **9** Difficulty **8** Solitude **2**
ROUND-TRIP DISTANCE	15 miles to Indian Bar; 16 miles to Cowlitz Park
ELEVATION GAIN	4000 feet to Indian Bar; 3900 feet to Cowlitz Park
OPTIONAL MAP	*Green Trails: Mount Rainier East*
USUALLY OPEN	Late July to October
BEST TIMES	Late July to October
AGENCY	Mount Rainier National Park
PERMIT	Required. Reservations are advised. All cars must also display an entry permit for the national park.
RESERVATION INFORMATION	Mount Rainier National Park sets aside only 40 percent of its available backcountry permits on a first-come, first-served basis. The remaining permits are given to hikers who made advance reservations. Since obtaining a permit for popular areas, especially on summer weekends, is extremely difficult, it is highly recommended that you reserve a permit in advance. Reservations are accepted starting on March 15 by mail, fax, or in person at the Longmire Wilderness Information Center. You cannot make a reservation over the phone. The cost is $20 per group and is nonrefundable. To obtain a reservation form and for further information, go to www.nps.gov/mora/planyourvisit/wilderness-reservation-information.htm.

Highlights

One of the classic beauty spots in Mount Rainier National Park, Indian Bar is a fairly small but spectacular basin of abundant wildflowers, streaking waterfalls, and outstanding mountain scenery. There may be no more beautiful location in the Pacific Northwest backcountry. Unfortunately, there are only a handful of designated backpacker campsites at Indian Bar, and the place is justifiably popular, so it can be very hard to get a permit. Apply for a reserved permit well in advance, although even then it helps to be lucky.

For those willing to put in the extra time and effort required to visit a cross-country area, however, there is another option. Not far southwest of Indian Bar sits the off-trail camping zone of Cowlitz Park, a rolling land of alpine meadows, wildflowers, and numerous waterfalls. Although Cowlitz Park is harder to reach, it actually has a better view of the mountain than does Indian Bar. Although it is usually possible to obtain a permit for Cowlitz Park, it is not a sure thing. The park currently allows only three parties a night to stay there, so it is often full as well, especially on weekends. Have an alternate plan in mind.

Getting There

Leave Interstate 5 north of Vancouver, Washington at Exit 68 and travel 72 miles east on U.S. Highway 12 to a junction with State Highway 123 about 7.5 miles past the town of Packwood. Turn left, following signs to Mount Rainier National Park, and drive a little over 5 miles to a junction with Stevens Canyon Road. Turn left, immediately passing through an entrance station for the park, and drive 10 miles to the Box Canyon Trailhead, just before a bridge over Muddy Fork Cowlitz River.

Hiking It

The trail departs from the north side of the road across from the parking lot and soon comes to a junction with the Wonderland Trail. It is worthwhile to turn left here and make a 0.2-mile side trip to check out Box Canyon, an extremely narrow cleft where the wa-

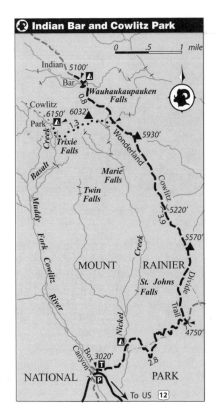

Indian Bar and Cowlitz Park

ters of the Muddy Fork Cowlitz River shoot through a steep-sided gorge.

After the short side trip, return to the junction and follow the Wonderland Trail as it gradually ascends a mostly forested hillside, and then loses a little elevation before coming to a bridged crossing of Nickel Creek at 0.8 mile. There is a designated backpacker camping area on the left. The sites here are pleasant, but the camp area has poor drainage, so it tends to turn into a shallow lake after a hard rain.

After crossing Nickel Creek you make a long, switchbacking, generally viewless climb that gains some 1500 feet in 2 miles to a junction with the Olallie Creek Trail at a wooded pass atop Cowlitz Divide. Keep left on the

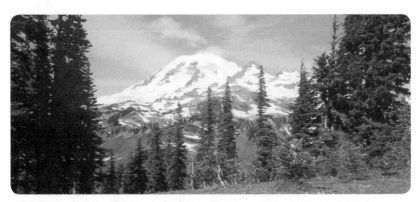

Mount Rainier from the Wonderland Trail on Cowlitz Divide, Mount Rainier National Park

Wonderland Trail and climb in forest for 1 mile to a grassy knoll where you gain the first really nice views of the hike. From this point you can see Mt. Rainier to the northwest as well as the rugged Cowlitz Chimneys to the north and down into the heavily forested Ohanapecosh Valley to the east. To the southwest is the jagged Tatoosh Range.

The trail's next section is wildly scenic as it descends to a saddle, and then goes up and down (mostly up), never straying far from the top of Cowlitz Divide. The route is a mix of meadows and partial forest with frequent views that continue to improve as you get closer to the park's massive, glacier-clad centerpiece. Wildlife is common in this area. Look for black bears, elk, deer, and a variety of mountain birds. At 6.1 miles you come to the top of a knoll where the views of Mt. Rainier are absolutely spectacular. With wildflowers in the foreground and trees framing the scene, this is one of the author's favorite spots to photograph the mountain. You can also look south to distant Mt. Adams. From the knoll, the trail makes a moderately steep descent, following a ridgeline to the

northwest for 0.4 mile before leveling out in a rolling meadow.

If you are headed for Cowlitz Park, leave the trail at this meadow and go left (almost due west) through mostly open, rolling terrain. The hiking isn't overly difficult, but as with all cross-country travel, your progress will be slower and more challenging than it was on trail. You soon cross two small creeks, and then ascend rather steeply on a mostly rocky slope before passing on the south side of a small knoll. Continue west, now on more level terrain, and make your way gradually uphill, going west-southwest for another 0.5 mile until you reach the drainage of Basalt Creek in the lower reaches of Cowlitz Park. On your left is a steep cliff over which creeks tumble in long drops. The most impressive of these cataracts is Trixie Falls on a small side stream feeding into Basalt Creek. Some of the best camps (there are no official or established sites in this off-trail zone) are along the lower reaches of the creek well above the cliffs. As always, choose a site well away from water and with a hard surface to avoid damaging the fragile alpine vegetation. You should expect to spend considerable time looking for a suitable site.

It is worthwhile to explore the upper reaches of Cowlitz Park to enjoy its fine views of Mt. Rainier and plentiful wildflowers.

If you have a permit to stay at Indian Bar, continue on the Wonderland Trail from the meadow where the Cowlitz Park route took off, and go downhill at a moderately steep grade until you come to the south end of Indian Bar. Just before the trail crosses the Ohanapecosh River, which here is only a creek, a trail goes left to a picturesque stone shelter. Camping here is generally restricted to groups of six or more people. The main trail crosses the "river" just above where the water plunges over thunderous Wauhaukaupauken Falls. Unfortunately it is almost as hard to get a good look at this falls as it is to spell the name. Immediately after the crossing, a signed trail goes to the right on its way to the designated campsites of Indian Bar.

After setting up camp, take the time to do a bit of exploring. At a minimum, walk up the Wonderland Trail across the lovely and amazingly flat expanse of Indian Bar, with its waving grasses, gravel beds, and acres of wildflowers. The surrounding cliffs and ridges that enclose the basin host several impressive but unnamed waterfalls on small creeks that drain from the permanent snowfields and small glacier above. If you have the energy for a longer adventure, continue on the Wonderland Trail as it ascends a ridge above the green expanse of Ohanapecosh Park, and then climbs over rocks and semipermanent snowfields to the views from Panhandle Gap, 3 miles from Indian Bar. Keep an eye out for wildlife, since Panhandle Gap is one of the better places in the park to see mountain goats.

WARNING

Although the route to Panhandle Gap is very scenic, the way is often covered with snow and difficult to follow before about mid-August.

7 Dumbbell and Sand Lakes Loop

RATINGS	Scenery **6** Difficulty **5** Solitude **6**
ROUND-TRIP DISTANCE	11.3 miles
ELEVATION GAIN	1550 feet
OPTIONAL MAP	*Green Trails: White Pass*
USUALLY OPEN	Mid-July to October
BEST TIMES	Late August to early September and early to mid-October
AGENCY	Naches Ranger District (Wenatchee National Forest)
PERMIT	None. Northwest Forest Pass required.

Highlights

The southern William O. Douglas Wilderness is a relatively gentle landscape of countless lakes, wonderful meadows, and attractive forests. Perhaps the area's most outstanding feature, however, becomes evident only from very late September through mid-October, when the millions of huckleberry bushes lining this area's lakes and meadows

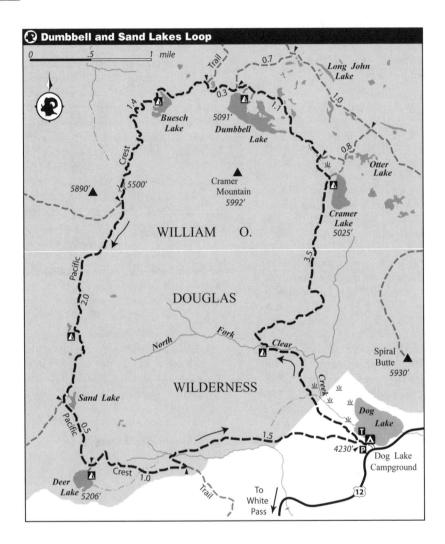

Dumbbell and Sand Lakes Loop

turn bright orange and red, putting on one of the better fall-color displays in our region. Fortuitously, this is also a time when crowds are few and the mosquitoes, which can be voracious in July and early August, are nearly gone. Late August to early September is also a nice time to visit, since the lakes are reasonably warm for swimming and you can feast on all those ripe huckleberries.

Getting There

Leave Interstate 5 north of Vancouver, Washington, at Exit 68 and travel 85 miles east on U.S. Highway 12 to White Pass. Continue east another 2.1 miles, then turn left into the signed DOG LAKE CAMPGROUND. The unpaved campground loop road passes the signed trailhead on the right after just 0.1 mile.

Hiking It

The trail starts in a relatively open mid-elevation forest of mixed conifers with plenty of huckleberries, fireweed, grouse whortleberries, and numerous other low-growing flowers and shrubs scattered about on the forest floor. After just 0.1 mile of uphill, the trail forks at the start of the loop.

Bear right onto the Cramer Lake Trail and follow this wide, horse-pounded path as it traces a very gentle course for 1.2 miles to a camp immediately before a bridgeless crossing of North Fork Clear Creek. There is usually a log you can scoot across here, but if that is missing, the creek crossing is an easy calf-deep ford.

After crossing the creek, the trail makes a gradual uphill traverse of a mostly forested hillside, and then turns north and wanders gently uphill to Cramer Lake at 3.2 miles. The trail stays in the forest, so far back from this good-sized and attractive lake that it is easy to walk right past it without noticing. The lake is worth a visit, however, so watch carefully and follow any of several sketchy trails that branch to the right and lead to this forest-rimmed gem. The lake has a fine campsite at its northwest end.

Just beyond Cramer Lake is a junction at the southeast corner of a lush grassy meadow. Watch for deer and elk here, especially early in the morning. This meadow is only the first of several forest-rimmed meadows you will visit over the next few miles. All of these meadows feature plenty of wildflowers in mid- to late July and bright red and orange huckleberry bushes in early October. Keep straight at the junction and walk around the southwest side of the small meadow, coming to a second

junction immediately after you cross a tiny creek. Turn left and climb a little more before catching a glimpse of large Dumbbell Lake. Unfortunately, this glimpse is all you will see of this scenic lake for some time as the trail stays in forest well back from the lake, instead passing several small but attractive ponds. After 0.4 mile you pass two unsigned but obvious use paths going to the left. These lead to campsites near the northwest end of Dumbbell Lake. Although well located, the camps are rather unattractive, since a recent fire killed many of the surrounding trees.

The main trail finally approaches Dumbbell Lake at its northwest tip,

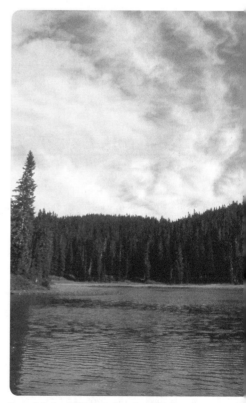

Buesch Lake, William O. Douglas Wilderness

where there is a signed junction with a very faint sign for Long John Trail. Go straight and follow a gentle path past more ponds and meadows for 0.3 mile to a junction with the Pacific Crest Trail (PCT). Turn left (southbound) on this wide and well-graded trail and walk 0.3 mile to beautiful, meadow-lined Buesch Lake. The trail skirts the north and west sides of the lake, passing a short side trail that leads to an exceptionally nice campsite above the west shore.

The PCT now climbs away from Buesch Lake, gradually ascending for 0.8 mile to a broad pass with two shallow ponds before coming to a signed junction with the faint Cortright Creek Trail. Keep straight on the PCT and go gradually up and down for 1.6 miles past tiny ponds and small meadows to a fine camp at a large and scenic pond just to the right (west) of the trail. From here you go downhill to a junction beside Sand Lake. The water in this lake recedes dramatically by late summer, reducing its attractiveness.

Keep left at the junction, still on the PCT, and after 0.6 mile come to a wide and heavily used side trail that goes to the right 80 yards to Deer Lake. There is a very large and comfortable camping area above this nearly circular lake's northeast shore.

The PCT continues east from Deer Lake, gradually losing elevation as it follows the hillside above the tiny outlet creek of Deer Lake. About 1.1 miles from the lake, you come to a junction where you turn sharply left on Dark Meadow Trail. After 0.1 mile this path crosses a tiny creek in a meadow, and then turns east and goes up and down for 0.5 mile before descending to the junction just above Dog Lake Campground and the close of the loop. Turn right to return to the trailhead.

8 | Cispus Point

RATINGS	Scenery **7** Difficulty **3** Solitude **9**
ROUND-TRIP DISTANCE	5.6 miles (with side trip)
ELEVATION GAIN	1400 feet
OPTIONAL MAP	*Green Trails: Blue Lake*
USUALLY OPEN	July to October
BEST TIMES	July
AGENCY	Cowlitz Valley Ranger District (Gifford Pinchot National Forest)
PERMIT	None

Highlights

This short but exciting hike takes you into a small but very attractive parcel of roadless terrain not far from Packwood, Washington. Since most hikers prefer the more famous trails around the scenic wonders of nearby Mt. Rainier and the Goat Rocks, it's not surprising that few people visit Cispus Point. Those who do are rewarded not only with solitude but with exceptional scenery, including plenty of views of those much more crowded attractions.

Getting There

Leave Interstate 5 north of Vancouver, Washington, at Exit 68 and travel 61 miles east on U.S. Highway 12 to an unsigned junction with Forest Road 20 near Milepost 127.6. Turn right (south) on this narrow and sometimes rough gravel road, staying on the main route at several minor intersections for 9.2 miles. Park at a pullout on the left about 0.2 mile past the signed trailhead for Jackpot Lake and just before the road leaves an old clear-cut.

Hiking It

The unsigned but obvious trail goes southwest along the edge of the clear-cut for 0.2 mile to a junction with the Klickitat Trail. Turn right and wander through a forest of mountain hemlocks and Alaska yellow cedars, which provide lots of welcome shade, but block most of the views. In July, wildflowers such as valerian, avalanche lily, columbine, wallflower, pink heather, bluebell, and lupine provide plenty of color, especially in places that get a bit more sun. Those breaks in the forest cover also provide views of bulky, snow-covered Mt. Adams to the south.

At 0.4 mile you begin an uphill traverse of an open rocky slope directly beneath the imposing cliffs on the east face of Cispus Point. The ascent ends at a junction in a small meadow with a shallow seasonal pond. Look for marsh marigolds and western anemones growing in the wet soils here.

The trail that goes left at this junction is the route to Cispus Point. Since this is such an easy hike, however, it is worth spending a little extra time and

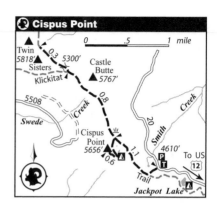

energy on a short side trip. So drop your pack and take the trail to the right, hiking mostly on the level through an open forest of subalpine firs and mountain hemlocks around the southwest side of massive Castle Butte. After 0.8 mile you come to a signed fork. The main Klickitat Trail goes left, but veer right, climb briefly to a saddle with a terrific view of Mt. Rainier, and then descend a little before turning north for a fun and scenic walk beneath the towering cliffs of Twin Sisters. This is the logical turnaround point for the side trip.

Back at the meadow junction, go south on the dead-end spur trail to Cispus Point, which climbs through forest then over open slopes before passing above a pair of small ponds with a couple of good and wildly scenic campsites. These camps are a bit exposed and the ponds are too shallow for either swimming or fishing, but they feature terrific views and plenty of solitude. The sunrises here can be spectacular. The trail continues past the pond, ascending to a ridgetop where it switchbacks to the right, and then climbs to the cliff-edged top of Cispus Point. The views here are outstanding and include all of the big volcanic peaks of southern Washington—Rainier, Adams, St. Helens, and

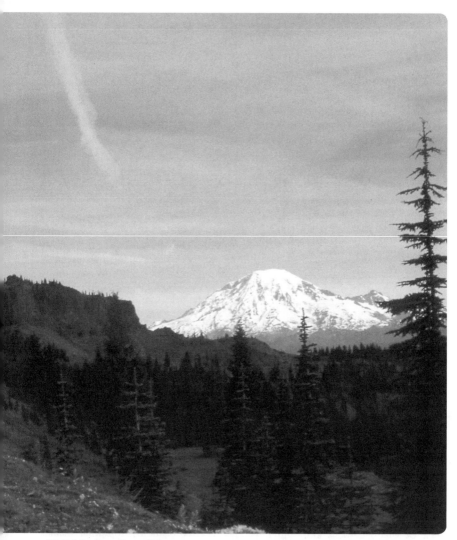

Mt. Rainier from Cispus Point

the eroded old volcano of the Goat Rocks. You can also look south to Oregon's Mt. Hood and see countless smaller rocky ridges and summits closer at hand. Sadly, several clear-cuts are also visible, but even they can't spoil a view that is this good.

9 Packwood Lake and Coyote Ridge Loop

RATINGS	Scenery **8** Difficulty **3 to 9** Solitude **2 to 8**
ROUND-TRIP DISTANCE	9 miles to Packwood Lake; 25.4 miles for loop
ELEVATION GAIN	300 feet to Packwood Lake; 4350 feet for loop
OPTIONAL MAPS	*Green Trails: Packwood, White Pass*
USUALLY OPEN	May to November for Packwood Lake; late July to October for loop
BEST TIMES	Late July to August
AGENCY	Cowlitz Valley Ranger District (Gifford Pinchot National Forest)
PERMIT	Required. Free at the trailhead. Northwest Forest Pass required.

to Packwood Lake

Highlights

Packwood Lake is a huge subalpine gem with a scenic island and terrific views up to the snowy crags of Johnson Peak. It is also accessible along an easy trail from a trailhead reached by a good paved road. Not surprisingly, the place is very popular. What many visitors don't realize, however, is that the lake is only the starting point for a magnificent backcountry loop. The trail along Coyote Ridge is one of the finest high-elevation ridge walks in our region, with outstanding views, plenty of wildlife, and abundant wildflowers. The amazing thing is that the ridge is so little traveled that you may have the entire route to yourself.

Getting There

Leave Interstate 5 north of Vancouver, Washington, at Exit 68 and travel 64 miles east on U.S. Highway 12 to the small town of Packwood. Near the north end of town, and immediately south of the Packwood Ranger Station/Work Center, turn right on Snyder Road, following signs to Packwood Lake Trail. This paved road, which becomes Forest Road 1260, climbs 3.8 miles to the large roadend parking lot and trailhead.

Hiking It

The heavily used trail departs from the north end of the parking lot and gently climbs under the shade of tall Douglas firs and western hemlocks. All that shade limits the understory to a few salal, Oregon grape, elderberry, thimbleberry, and scattered forest wildflowers. The next 4.2 miles are easy hiking with very little elevation gain or loss, staying in generally viewless but pleasant forest. At the end of this section you descend a little to the west shore of very large and green-tinged Packwood Lake. This photogenic lake, with its large, forested island and views of Johnson Peak, is the destination of almost all hikers, so beyond this point you will enjoy much more solitude.

The trail passes a relatively new guard station building just before a signed junction with the Pipeline Trail, an old road that parallels the hiker's trail and is often used by mountain bikers and motorcyclists to access the

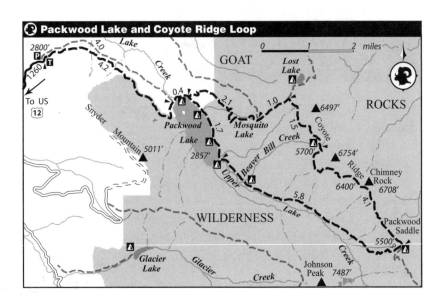

Packwood Lake and Coyote Ridge Loop

lake. Shortly after this junction your trail passes the historic 1910 log ranger station building and then takes a bridge over the lake's dammed outlet creek. Shortly after this crossing are some fine campsites, featuring excellent views to the southeast of Johnson Peak rising over the waters of Packwood Lake.

At 4.6 miles the trail forks at the start of the recommended loop. Veer left (uphill) and immediately pull away from the lake as the trail steadily climbs at a moderately steep grade across a heavily forested hillside. The circuitous route ascends in switchbacks and winding traverses for 2 miles before reaching a tiny, lily-pad-covered pond that goes by the name of Mosquito Lake. Although this is not much of a "lake," it does feature a decent campsite above its northwest shore.

The trail rounds the west and north sides of Mosquito Lake, and then continues 0.1 mile to an easy-to-miss junction. Stay straight on the main trail and contour for 0.4 mile to a lovely wildflower meadow before climbing in forest for 0.6 mile to a junction.

Veer right (uphill) on Coyote Ridge Trail and continue a steady uphill as the forest becomes more open, with mountain hemlocks, subalpine firs, Alaska yellow cedars, and other high-elevation trees replacing the lower elevation types you saw earlier in the trip. At 9.2 miles you reach a fine campsite next to small Beaver Bill Creek, the last campsite and the last reliable water for several miles.

Beyond Beaver Bill Creek the trail ascends 300 feet to round the end of a ridge with great views of Mt. Rainier to the northwest, and then settles into a pattern of ups and downs along the southwest side of Coyote Ridge. The scenery for the next 4 miles is stupendous, with views south to Mt. St. Helens, down to Packwood Lake, and across the canyon to the snowy and jagged pinnacles of Johnson Peak and Old Snowy Mountain. Add to these distant vistas the fine, close-up views of impressive Chimney Rock, which sits atop Coyote Ridge, and you have a real winner. Wildlife is common as well. Look for pikas, elk, deer, and black bears, along with a wide variety of mountain birds. And don't forget the wildflowers! The mostly open slopes here are carpeted with flowers throughout the summer. A partial list of species includes bellflower, spiraea, beargrass, lupine, aster, pearly everlasting, false hellebore, buckwheat, partridgefoot, yarrow, bistort, and paintbrush. On the downside, the trail is narrow and eroded in places, so be careful where you step.

The trail reaches its highest point when it tops Coyote Ridge on the southeast side of Chimney Rock. From here you go steeply downhill on a narrow, gravel-strewn route, losing almost 900 feet to a junction at Packwood Saddle. There is a small campsite near this junction with water available from a spring about 0.2 mile down the trail to the right.

The recommended loop trail goes right (downhill) from Packwood Saddle, but if you have the time and energy it is worth taking a side trip that goes straight and climbs for a little less than 1 mile to an extremely photogenic viewpoint on the shoulder of Egg Butte. The scene looking back down the length of rugged Coyote Ridge to the glacier-covered summit of Mt. Rainier is outstanding. This is also a good place to look for mountain goats, the animals that gave the Goat Rocks Wilderness its name.

Back at Packwood Saddle, turn west and descend steeply through dense forest past a spring and across several tiny creeks as you steadily lose elevation. The downhill continues for 2.5 miles before finally bottoming out back in lower-elevation forest along Upper Lake Creek. From here the trail turns downstream, doing only minor ups and downs for the next several miles as it follows the meandering

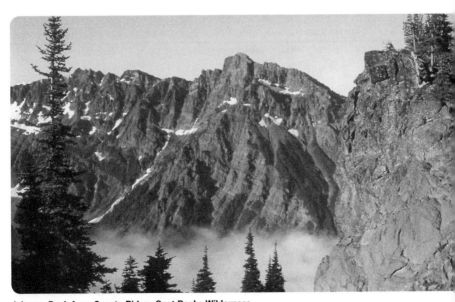

Johnson Peak from Coyote Ridge, Goat Rocks Wilderness

creek. The walk would be easy, except that in late 2006 a major flood hit this area, changing the course of the creek in several places, leaving behind numerous washouts, and killing many of the trees. Most of the route is in good shape, but you'll still have to scramble around washouts in a couple of spots and watch for cairns where the flood waters obliterated the tread. The best place to camp is at 18.5 miles, immediately after you cross the lower end of Beaver Bill Creek.

About 0.6 mile of up and down past Beaver Bill Creek takes you to an invit-ing campsite at the southeast end of Packwood Lake. This camp features a good if partially obstructed view of Mt. Rainier and offers the camper a chance to see ospreys flying over the lake. The camps at this end of the lake are much less crowded than those along the more easily accessible north shore. The trail goes around the east side of Packwood Lake, offering many fine views of this large, deep, and very scenic lake and passing a half dozen possible campsites to a junction at the close of the loop at 20.8 miles. Go straight and return the way you came.

10 Heart Lake

RATINGS	Scenery **8** Difficulty **7** Solitude **6**
ROUND-TRIP DISTANCE	13.4 miles
ELEVATION GAIN	2400 feet
OPTIONAL MAP	*Green Trails*: *Blue Lake*
USUALLY OPEN	Late July to October
BEST TIMES	Late July to October
AGENCY	Cowlitz Valley Ranger District (Gifford Pinchot National Forest)
PERMIT	Required. Free at the trailhead.

Highlights

This relatively uncrowded trail samples all of the many charms of the Goat Rocks Wilderness. Starting in a lovely high-elevation forest, you ascend into flower-choked meadows along a ridge with amazing views of Packwood Lake and Mt. Rainier, pass through a rocky basin below craggy Johnson Peak, and then descend to gorgeous Heart Lake in a scenic basin beneath meadowy slopes. Best of all the lake features a wonderful campsite in a grove of trees with fine views and surprisingly few people.

Getting There

Leave Interstate 5 north of Vancouver, Washington, at Exit 68 and travel 63 miles east on U.S. Highway 12 to a poorly signed junction with Forest Road 48 near Milepost 129.5. Turn right on this initially good gravel road, remaining on the main route and ignoring several minor intersections as the road steadily climbs. The road gets rough and quite steep in one spot just beyond a gravel pit, but if your vehicle has decent ground clearance you should have no problem. The trailhead is on the right, 11.2 miles from Highway 12.

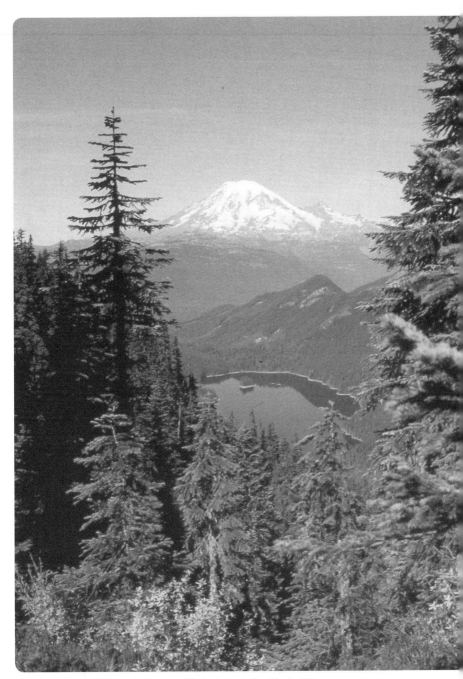

Mount Rainier and Packwood Lake from Lily Basin Trail, Goat Rocks Wilderness

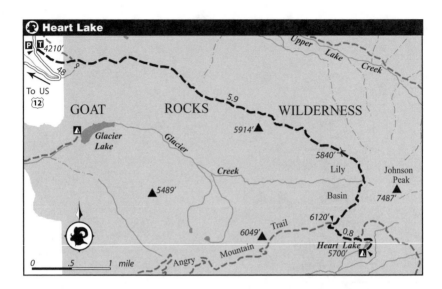

There is a small parking area about 30 yards past the trailhead.

Hiking It

The Lily Basin Trail begins with a steady climb through a lovely forest of Douglas firs, western hemlocks, and Pacific silver firs, with an understory of beargrass and huckleberries. At 0.6 mile a horse trail splits off to the left. Go straight, still climbing, through a pleasant but generally viewless forest, and at about 1 mile begin following a wooded ridgeline.

As you traverse the north side of the ridge at about 3.5 miles, you hit the first of several breaks in the tree cover that reveal spectacularly photogenic views to the northeast of Mt. Rainier with Packwood Lake and its distinctive island in the foreground below. At 4.3 miles you cross through a little saddle onto the south side of the ridge and enjoy good views of rugged Johnson Peak about 1 mile to the southeast.

After working its way to the east, the up-and-down trail cuts across the steep, rocky, and mostly open slopes on the west side of Johnson Peak above forested Lily Basin. Tiny creeks here provide the first water of the trip. There are fine views along this section, both of the forested canyon to the west and of imposing Johnson Peak to the east. The trail eventually climbs to the top of a ridge on the southwest side of Johnson Peak, where you enjoy terrific views to the southwest of Mt. St. Helens, northwest to Mt. Rainier, and south to a small part of Mt. Adams. There is also a junction here with the Angry Mountain Trail.

You veer left (downhill) at the junction, make one quick switchback, and then make a downhill traverse of a partly forested slope for 0.6 mile to an unsigned fork with the spur trail to Heart Lake. Turn right and descend 0.2 mile to the lovely green-tinged pool, which is surrounded by meadows and backed by scenic ridges. There are excellent camps near the outlet at the lake's west end.

11 Snowgrass Flat Loop

RATINGS	Scenery **10** Difficulty **6** Solitude **1**
ROUND-TRIP DISTANCE	14.3 miles (with many great side trip options)
ELEVATION GAIN	3000 feet
OPTIONAL MAP	*U.S. Forest Service: Goat Rocks Wilderness*
USUALLY OPEN	Late July to October
BEST TIMES	Late July through August
AGENCY	Cowlitz Valley Ranger District (Gifford Pinchot National Forest)
PERMIT	Required. Free at the trailhead. Northwest Forest Pass required.

Highlights

The sloping, flower-covered meadows of Snowgrass Flat are one of the most popular hiking destinations in Washington, and with good reason, because this is without question one of the premier hikes in the Pacific Northwest. The scenery is outstanding, with plenty of views of rugged mountains both near and far, a stunning glacial lake, thousands of acres of wildflowers, numerous scenic campsites, and gorgeous alpine ridges. If you like mountain scenery, then this country is beyond compare. It is highly recommended, however, that you time your visit for a weekday to make the crowd situation more tolerable.

Getting There

Leave Interstate 5 north of Vancouver, Washington, at Exit 68 and travel 62 miles east on U.S. Highway 12 to a signed junction with Forest Road 21 near Milepost 128.4. Turn right (south), following signs to Chambers Lake, and stay on this good gravel road for 13.4 miles to a junction. Turn left on Road 2150, drive 3 miles, and then veer right at a fork. Proceed 0.1 mile to a junction, go right on the trailhead loop road, and continue 0.4 mile to the scattered parking along the road for the popular Snowgrass Trailhead.

Hiking It

You begin in a relatively open mid-elevation forest of mixed conifers with an unusually high concentration of huckleberries and beargrass carpeting the forest floor. After just 0.1 mile there is a junction at the start of the loop. For the recommended clockwise circuit, go sharply left on a horse trail, which soon passes a marshy lake before making a 0.3-mile traverse through forest and small wildflower meadows to a junction just 10 yards from a secondary trailhead.

You turn right onto the Goat Ridge Trail and immediately begin a steady uphill, with the vegetation changing to the usual higher-elevation varieties as you ascend. At 1.7 miles go straight at a junction with an alternate side loop trail, and then climb a little more to a nice viewpoint looking east to the jagged summits of the Goat Rocks. From here you descend to a saddle and a reunion with the alternate loop trail.

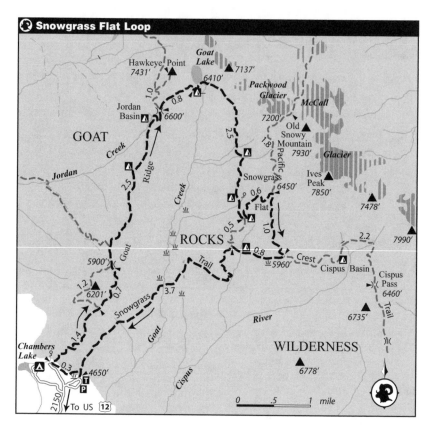

Snowgrass Flat Loop

Your trail goes straight, crosses to the west side of Goat Ridge, and then makes an up-and-down traverse with partial views looking north-northwest to Mt. Rainier. You pass a junction with the faint Jordan Creek Trail, and then go up and down across a partially forested hillside that features several sloping wildflower meadows. From late July to mid-August the color show is terrific. Look for lupine, aster, columbine, pearly everlasting, yarrow, western anemone, bistort, pink heather, false hellebore, arnica, groundsel, cat's ear, and a dozen other species. At 3.6 miles you pass a grandly scenic campsite on a knoll on the left side of the trail. This camp features outstanding

views of the nearby ridges and canyons as well as distant Mt. St. Helens. Unfortunately, the only nearby water is from seasonal trickles of snowmelt that are usually gone by late summer.

The trail now rounds a huge sloping basin beneath a scenic ridge, and then climbs into Jordan Basin, which has reliable water, grandly scenic but exposed camps, and a (really) small pond. From here the trail climbs a pair of switchbacks to a 6600-foot pass and a junction with Lily Basin Trail. A wonderful side trip from here goes left for 0.4 mile, then right on the trail to the top of Hawkeye Point. Views from this summit extend to almost every major landmark for more than 50 miles.

You veer right and make a wildly scenic traverse of an open slope with several small trickling creeks. This slope, which is a sea of wildflowers in late summer, features breathtaking views of Mt. Adams to the south and east to Snowgrass Flat and the Goat Rocks crest. At the northeast end of the traverse, the trail descends to Goat Lake, a milky gem (the color comes from glacial silt) that is usually covered with ice until sometime in August. This scenic pool has good but exposed camps and an awesome setting beneath stark, rocky slopes and snowfields. Campfires are prohibited within 0.25 mile of the lake.

The trail crosses the lake's outlet creek well above an unseen sloping waterfall, and then contours across open slopes before entering the lower portion of Snowgrass Flat. This alpine paradise is a wonderland of scattered tree islands, bubbling creeks, great campsites, and profuse wildflowers. The trail goes up and down for a little over 1 mile through this gorgeous meadowland before coming to an area with a confusion of trails, most of which soon dead-end at campsites. Veer left at the first major unsigned fork and, 150 yards later, reach a signed junction with Snowgrass Trail. Several trails converge here, but the unsigned ones are just dead-ends that lead to campsites.

The fastest way back to the trailhead is to turn right on the Snowgrass Trail, but to visit the spectacular upper part of Snowgrass Flat you should turn left and climb a series of lazy switchbacks to the flower-covered upper meadows and a junction with the Pacific Crest Trail (PCT). Great views are almost as

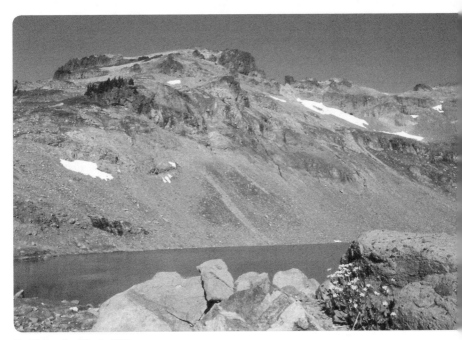

Goat Lake, Goat Rocks Wilderness

common as the flowers here, with fine vistas south to Mt. Adams and east to the nearby jagged summits of Ives Peak, Old Snowy Mountain, and a host of unnamed summits along the crest of the Goat Rocks. The whole area is a photographer's delight. Turning left (north) at the junction with the PCT will soon take you into above-timberline terrain and lead to miles of scenic hiking all the way to a ridgetop viewpoint just above Packwood Glacier. To loop back, however, you should turn right (south) on the PCT and descend through more lovely meadows for 1 mile to a large cairn marking the junction with Bypass Trail. For a great side trip from here, continue straight (southbound) on the PCT for 1 mile to scenic Cispus Basin, and then hike another mile up to the views from Cispus Pass.

The recommended loop goes sharply right at the junction onto the Bypass Trail, which goes downhill through forest to a hop-over crossing of a lovely creek. There are some good campsites at this crossing. Just 0.2 mile past this creek is a junction with Snowgrass Trail. Turn left and soon descend a series of well-graded switchbacks. From the bottom of these switchbacks make a gentle, woodsy walk to a bridged crossing of Goat Creek, and then climb briefly before making a 1-mile contour across a forested hillside back to the junction 0.1 mile from the trailhead. Keep left to return to your car.

Mount Saint Helens and Vicinity

Our world-famous resident volcano, Mt. St. Helens, proved in the spring and summer of 1980 the dangers of having unresolved anger issues. In May of that year she released 123 years of pent-up frustrations by literally blowing her top (over 1300 feet of which simply disappeared) and turning everything for a dozen miles or so to the north into a scorched wasteland. Although this event put a damper on her previous considerable beauty, if anything it seems to have increased her appeal, because ever since her (not so) little outburst people have been flocking to her doorstep to take in the view and see how the neighborhood is recovering. And that is understandable, because exploring this fascinating and strangely compelling landscape is like no other hiking experience in North America. Fortunately, the Forest Service, which oversees the national volcanic monument, has developed a network of exciting hiking trails where hikers and backpackers can enjoy the scenery at a pace that car-bound tourists can never fully appreciate. If the volcanic landscape isn't to your liking, the area just south and southeast of the mountain holds some superb trails that explore scenic canyons filled with clear streams, waterfalls, and old-growth forests.

12 Dome Camp

RATINGS	Scenery **9** Difficulty **6** Solitude **3**
ROUND-TRIP DISTANCE	14.2 miles
ELEVATION GAIN	1950 feet
OPTIONAL MAP	*Green Trails: Mount St. Helens*
USUALLY OPEN	Mid-June to October
BEST TIMES	Late June to mid-July
AGENCY	Mount St. Helens National Volcanic Monument
PERMIT	Required. Free, but reservations are strongly advised. Northwest Forest Pass required.
RESERVATION INFORMATION	Backcountry camping permits are required for spending the night in the Mt. Margaret Backcountry. Advance reservations are strongly encouraged, as the camps are very popular during the summer. There is no fee for the reservation or the permit, but you must have a Northwest Forest Pass to obtain a permit. Reservations may be made by mail, fax, or in person at the monument headquarters. You cannot make a reservation over the phone. To obtain a reservation form and the all other necessary information go to www.fs.fed.us/gpnf/04mshnvm/backcountry/.

Highlights

The vast majority of the trails in the Pacific Northwest travel through miles of dense coniferous forests before ending at some ridge, lake, or other destination where you break out of the trees and can enjoy the view. In another 50 years or so that will probably be true of this hike as well. For now, though, this trail is a wonderfully open ramble with grand views, lots of wildflowers, and only a handful of scattered fir trees. This unusual scenery results from the dramatic handiwork of Mt. St. Helens, which fills the skyline just a few miles to the southeast. On the cataclysmic morning of May 18, 1980, the volcano flattened the forests and generally destroyed this entire area in one of the largest natural disasters in U.S. history. Walking through this recovering devastated area is a hiking experience unlike anything in North America.

WARNING

Volcanic activity is ongoing at Mt. St. Helens and is intermittently dangerous. In addition, this area's soft and unstable volcanic soils, with very little vegetation to hold them in place, make erosion and trail washouts a continuing problem. Trail closures for both reasons are common and may last for months. Check on current conditions before you travel here, so you don't waste a trip.

Water is scarce to nonexistent on this hike, and there are almost no trees to provide shade or protection from the wind. Be sure to carry extra water, sunglasses, a hat, and a windbreaker.

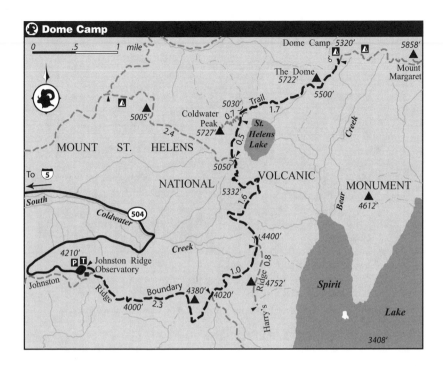

NOTE

To protect this fragile and scientifically important area, all off-trail travel (even by a few feet) is prohibited.

Getting There

Leave Interstate 5 north of Vancouver at Castle Rock Exit 49, following signs to Mount St. Helens National Volcanic Monument, and drive east on State Highway 504. Stay on this paved highway for almost 44 miles, then veer right at a fork and proceed 9.1 miles to the huge road-end parking lot for the Johnston Ridge Observatory and Visitors Center.

Hiking It

The initially paved, hiker-only trail departs from a large signboard at the northeast end of the parking lot. Vegetation is slowly reclaiming the surroundings. Look for willows, Sitka alders, a few scattered Pacific silver firs (now up to 20 feet tall), lupine, yarrow, pearly everlasting, wild strawberry, cliff penstemon, fireweed, and various other shrubs, grasses, and wildflowers. Look for them, that is, if you can take your eyes off the views of the mountain and the wildly eroded mudflows of the devastated area below.

After 100 yards the paved trail curves to the right on its way to the observatory, but you turn left on a gravelly path that goes gradually downhill. Careful inspection reveals that this "gravel" is actually a thick layer of pumice and coarse ash dropped by the volcano. Although this environment looks like a difficult place for animals to survive, keep an eye out for elk. Herds of 40 or more are fairly common, especially early in the morning.

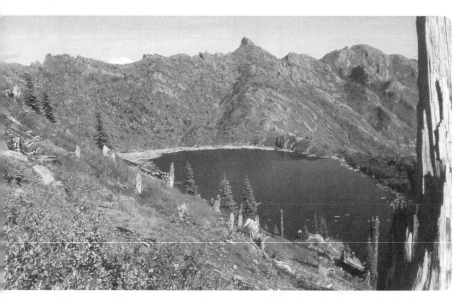

Peaks of Mount Margaret area over St. Helens Lake, Mount St. Helens National Volcanic Monument

Binoculars will help you get a better look.

After 0.8 mile the trail, which has been mostly downhill until now, changes to an up-and-down route along an open, undulating ridge. Views of the mountain are frequent and you can also see northeast to Coldwater Peak and some of the higher summits in the Mt. Margaret Backcountry. The trail makes a turn to the right (south) to go around a prominent high point, taking you to yet another fine view of the volcano at the end of the ridge. From here you can also see east for the first time to distant Mt. Adams and down to log-choked Spirit Lake.

At 2.3 miles you go straight on the Boundary Trail at the junction with Truman Trail and wind mostly uphill through a particularly erosion-prone area where posts have been installed to help you locate the correct route. At 3.3 miles is a junction. Harry's Ridge Trail goes right 0.8 mile before dead-ending

at yet another breathtaking viewpoint, this time featuring a particularly good perspective of Spirit Lake. Go left, still on the Boundary Trail, and steadily climb eight rather long switchbacks to the top of a ridge. From here you gain terrific, far-ranging views that include those looking south to Oregon's Mt. Hood as well as north to Mt. Rainier and the Goat Rocks. Deep, log-strewn St. Helens Lake sits in a basin between you and the rugged peaks of the Mt. Margaret area.

The now narrow and rugged trail descends two short switchbacks before passing through a natural rock arch and going up and down along the side of a ridge to a junction in a saddle on the south side of prominent Coldwater Peak. The Coldwater Trail goes left, but you go straight on the Boundary Trail, which crosses the steep slope on the east side of Coldwater Peak well above St. Helens Lake.

At 5.4 miles is a junction with the 0.7-mile side trail that switchbacks up to the top of Coldwater Peak. Go straight, soon pass through another saddle, and then curve to the right (east), crossing a slope well above the north shore of St. Helens Lake. Atop the ridge on your left are some impressively jagged rock formations. This stretch of trail also features some outstanding wildflower displays, especially of lupine. The show usually peaks sometime between late June and mid-July. The trail makes a final 500-foot climb to a high point on the south side

of The Dome, a prominent rocky peak, before descending to the signed turnoff to Dome Camp at 7.1 miles. Situated high on a ridge just northeast of The Dome, this scenic camp boasts 3 designated tent sites and grand views. The only water is from a tiny spring near the lower designated campsite not far from the roofless outhouse. The spring is usually reliable, but may stop flowing by late summer in particularly dry years. If the sites at Dome Camp are already taken, try to get a permit for Mt. Margaret Camp, another 0.5 mile to the east along the Boundary Trail.

13 Goat Mountain and Green River Loop

RATINGS	Scenery **7** Difficulty **8** Solitude **8**
ROUND-TRIP DISTANCE	17.9 miles
ELEVATION GAIN	3700 feet
OPTIONAL MAP	*Green Trails*: *Mount St. Helens*
USUALLY OPEN	Late June to October
BEST TIMES	Early July
AGENCY	Mount St. Helens National Volcanic Monument
PERMIT	None

Highlights
In the northern part of the Mount St. Helens National Volcanic Monument, only a few miles but seemingly a world away from the crowds that gather near the volcano, this wonderful loop hike explores the edge of the volcano's recovering devastated area. The loop has it all: high ridges with outstanding views; a mountain lake that is ideal for swimming; a lush river valley with huge old-growth forests; and, most surprisingly, very few people. In fact, the trails are more commonly used by

equestrians than by hikers. Despite the horses, the trails are in good shape and not badly damaged by hooves or overly aromatic from "apples."

Getting There
Leave Interstate 5 north of Vancouver, Washington, at Woodland Exit 21 and travel 23.5 miles east on Highway 503 to a junction. Go straight on Highway 503 Spur and proceed 24.2 miles to a junction immediately past the Pine Creek Information Station. Go straight, now on Forest Road 25, and drive 25.6

Goat Mountain and Green River Loop

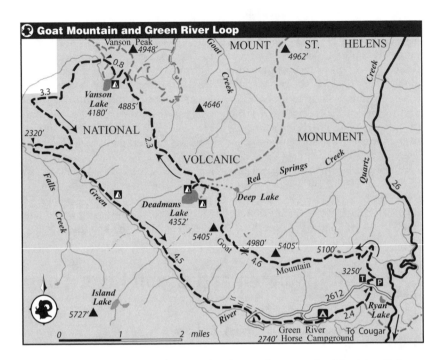

miles to a major intersection. Turn left on Road 99, following signs to Windy Ridge, go 9.2 miles, and then turn right on single-lane paved Road 26. In recent years this road has often been closed due to washouts. Call ahead for the latest conditions. Proceed 4.6 miles to a junction about 100 yards after the turnoff into the Ryan Lake Interpretive Site. Turn left on gravel Road 2612 and drive 0.4 mile to a large gravel trailhead parking lot on the right.

Hiking It

The trail begins from the west end of the parking lot and winds uphill at a moderately steep grade through an old clear-cut now populated by 20-foot-tall Douglas firs, western hemlocks, Pacific silver firs, western white pines, and Engelmann spruces. The sun can be oppressive here on hot summer days,

but it also provides life-giving light to many wildflowers, including Queen Anne's lace, penstemon, paintbrush, lousewort, and wild rose. Wildlife is also common. Look for elk, deer, black bear, coyote, ruffed and blue grouse, and various small birds.

At 1 mile the trail enters a pristine forest and you enjoy shade while you continue climbing. At 1.8 miles you reach the end of a ridgeline, make a sharp left turn, and then continue up-hill in a lichen-draped forest. About 0.5 mile and four short switchbacks later you leave the forest and finally enter the enchanting world atop Goat Mountain Ridge. This ridge is on the edge of the devastated area, so the forests on the north side of the ridge survived, while those to the south were killed by clouds of fast-moving super-heated gas. Two factors have allowed this area to recover more quickly than places nearer the volcano: first, plants had a shorter distance to go to recolonize the area; and second, the ground this far from the mountain was not completely sterilized by the searing heat, so some seeds managed to survive and sprout shortly after the eruption. As a result, wildflowers now abound in the meadows atop the ridge, including such colorful varieties as yarrow, lupine, wild strawberry, buckwheat, larkspur, and lomatium. Small trees have also colonized the ridgetop, adding to the scenery. But even with all the interesting geology and botany, it is the views that are this area's biggest attraction. Most impressive is the vista to the south over the deep chasm of the Green River Valley to the rugged snowy crags of the Mt. Margaret Backcountry. Rising behind these crags are the dramatic gray-streaked walls of the steaming crater of Mt. St. Helens. If you can pry your admiring eyes away from this scene, take a look to the north to massive Mt. Rainier, south to pointed Mt. Hood, and east to bulky Mt. Adams, each ominously awaiting its own inevitable opportunity to create volcanic mayhem.

For the next 1.5 miles the trail goes up and down near the top of the ridge, providing nonstop spectacular views. Near the western end of the traverse you cut across the south side of a ruggedly scenic high point on the ridge, and then drop to a saddle. From here you enjoy your last good view to the south of the devastated area and the Mt. Margaret Backcountry. The pass also supports some of the best flower fields along the entire loop.

From the saddle the trail steadily descends a brushy slope on the north side of the ridge, then enters forest and at about 4.5 miles passes a pair of unsigned but obvious junctions with side trails to campsites on Deadmans Lake. This lovely, forest-rimmed lake has a unique sandy shoreline that resulted from huge quantities of ash and pumice dropping here during the eruption. The resulting "beach" provides a fun way to wade out into the deeper water for a swim.

Just beyond Deadmans Lake the main trail comes to a junction with the Tumwater Mountain Trail. Go straight and follow a roller coaster route along a woodsy ridge. The vegetation is primarily open forests of subalpine and other true firs mixed with western white and lodgepole pines. Views are limited to a few glimpses of Mt. Rainier to the north, but the flowers are abundant, especially in late June and early July.

About 2.4 miles from Deadmans Lake is a four-way junction. Take the downhill trail to the left, and descend two rather steep switchbacks to a poorly marked junction. The trail to the left drops steeply to a campsite on the northeast shore of Vanson Lake. This is a nice spot, although the camping here is not as good as at Deadmans Lake. The main trail goes straight, descends to a junction with another spur to Vanson Lake, and soon reaches yet another trail junction. You go left, cross a small creek below a pretty little meadow, and then descend steadily through forest for 3.2 miles to a junction with the Green River Trail.

Turn left (east) on the Green River Trail and follow this joyful low-elevation route as it slowly ascends through an impressive old-growth forest of towering Douglas firs, never far from the clear water of misnamed Green River. After 1.4 miles you pass a pair of fine riverside campsites. Elk tracks and droppings are abundant in this area, so keep an eye out for these animals as you hike. Shortly after the campsites you

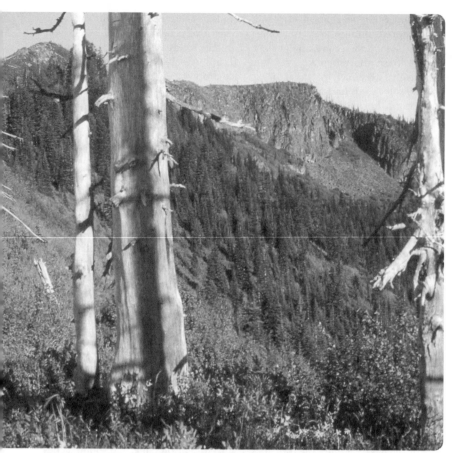

Goat Mountain Ridge from Goat Mountain Saddle, Mount St. Helens National Volcanic Monument

take a dilapidated wooden bridge over a side creek, and then go up and down for 0.6 mile before leaving the forest and entering the recovering devastated area. Tall snags left behind by the blast frame sweeping views both up to Goat Mountain Ridge on your left and of the many waterfalls on creeks dropping into the canyon from the peaks and lakes of the Mt. Margaret Backcountry on your right. Young fir trees are returning to this zone, but they have a long way to go to match the big old trees you passed farther downstream.

The wildflowers, however, are making a more rapid recovery, with plenty of bunchberry, lupine, columbine, daisy, spiraea, and other species colonizing the area.

At 15.5 miles you cross a gravel road, and then gradually make your way upstream through the devastated area to the Green River Horse Campground. The trail skirts the camp area, and then climbs more noticeably, passing a junction with a trail going to the right before returning to the trailhead.

14 Mount Margaret Backcountry Lakes

RATINGS	Scenery **8** Difficulty **6** Solitude **4**
ROUND-TRIP DISTANCE	12.2 miles to Panhandle Lake; 15.8 miles to pass above Shovel Lake
ELEVATION GAIN	2400 feet to Panhandle Lake; 3100 feet to pass above Shovel Lake
OPTIONAL MAP	*Green Trails: Mount St. Helens*
USUALLY OPEN	July to October
BEST TIMES	Mid- to late July
AGENCY	Mount St. Helens National Volcanic Monument
PERMIT	Required. Reservations are strongly advised. Northwest Forest Pass required.
RESERVATION INFORMATION	Backcountry camping permits are required for spending the night in the Mt. Margaret Backcountry. Advance reservations are strongly encouraged, as the camps are very popular during the summer. There is no fee for the reservation or the permit, but you must have a Northwest Forest Pass to obtain a permit. Reservations may be made by mail, fax, or in person at the monument headquarters. You cannot make a reservation over the phone. To obtain a reservation form and the all other necessary information go to www.fs.fed.us/gpnf/04mshnvm/backcountry/.

Highlights

The Mount Margaret Backcountry is a very scenic area in the rugged peaks north of Spirit Lake, filled with attractive mountain lakes, rocky peaks, flower fields, and great viewpoints. The region has been a popular hiking destination for decades, although its character changed dramatically (to use a woefully inadequate word) on May 18, 1980, when Mt. Margaret's larger and more hot-headed neighbor literally blew her stack, blasted out the world's largest clear-cut, and obliterated the entire neighborhood. Slowly, vegetation and trails are returning to this region providing hiking opportunities that are scenic and fascinating from both a botanical and a geologic point of view. To protect the fragile environment, all off-trail travel is prohibited and hikers are allowed to camp only at designated sites.

Getting There

Leave Interstate 5 north of Vancouver, Washington, at Woodland Exit 21 and travel 23.5 miles east on Highway 503 to a junction. Go straight on Highway 503 Spur and proceed 24.2 miles to a junction immediately past the Pine Creek Information Station. Go straight, now on Forest Road 25, and drive 25.6 miles to a major intersection. Turn left on Road 99, following signs to Windy Ridge, go 9.2 miles, and then turn right on Road 26. Drive 0.9 mile, then turn left into the large parking lot at the Norway Pass Trailhead.

Hiking It

The trail begins from the north side of the parking lot, soon crosses a little creek, and then goes gradually uphill through a landscape that continues to recover from the 1980 blast. In addition

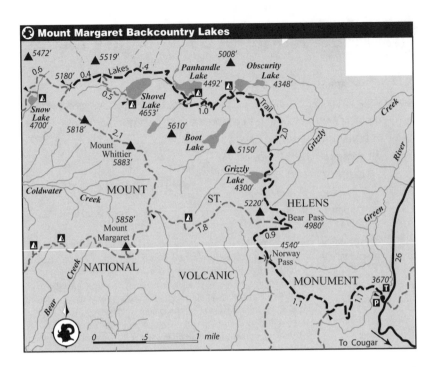

Mount Margaret Backcountry Lakes

to the obvious lack of big trees, evidence of the eruption comes in the form of countless downed logs and sand on the trail. Careful analysis reveals that the substance isn't really sand, but a mix of fine-grained ash and pumice, several feet of which fell here during the eruption. Various shrubs, including snowberries, huckleberries, and willows now grow atop this "sandy" material along with scattered wildflowers. Some of the more common blossoms include yarrow, fireweed, pearly everlasting, paintbrush, groundsel, and cliff penstemon. The few trees are mostly Pacific silver firs with some western hemlocks and Douglas firs. Although some of the trees are now over 20 feet tall, they remain few and far between, putting shade at a premium. Water is also rare, so bring plenty.

At 1.1 miles is a junction. Go right, climb a little more to the top of a small spur ridge, and then make a mostly level traverse to Norway Pass and a junction with the Independence Pass Trail. Here Mt. St. Helens rather suddenly makes her appearance on stage, and like any great performer she really steals the show. The gaping crater, which often emits an ominous cloud of steam, is on full display, as is the huge (and still growing) lava dome that now fills most of the crater.

Between you and the volcano sits Spirit Lake, still choked with millions of floating logs. The logs are the result of trees that were instantly killed and toppled by a fast-moving cloud of superheated gas. The dead logs were then swept back into the lake by an enormous avalanche-produced wave of water out of the lake. The scene is like nothing else in North America, and produces memories that are likely to last a lifetime.

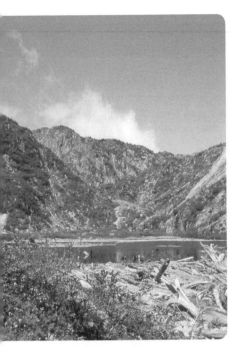

Grizzly Lake, Mount St. Helens National Volcanic Monument

After several minutes (or hours) of gaping in awe, go right at the junction and wind your way uphill to a junction at 3.1 miles. Turn right on Lakes Trail #211 and ascend 0.1 mile to a viewpoint at Bear Pass. From here the previously described view of Mt. St. Helens is joined by views of two older volcanoes, Mt. Adams to the east and Mt. Rainier to the north.

To reach the lakes, descend at a moderately steep grade on a narrow and often dangerously eroded trail that winds across a steep hillside, over little ridges, and past massive deadfall for 0.8 mile to Grizzly Lake. This deep and lovely lake is set in a steep-walled cirque basin and is surrounded (as are all lakes in this devastated region) by regrowing shrubs, downed logs, and a few young trees. Alpine wildflowers are

regaining a foothold here, especially pink heather and white partridgefoot. Like a smaller version of Spirit Lake, many logs float on the waters of Grizzly Lake. To the west rise steep slopes and cliffs that are still largely devoid of trees. It is a dramatic spot, and one that is well worth taking some time to admire, although camping is not allowed.

Cross the lake's outlet creek and then make a mile-long sidehill traverse with lots of minor ups and downs to Obscurity Lake, which is backed by a small, unnamed rocky butte to the northwest. A short spur trail leads to a cluster of designated campsites along the inlet creek at the lake's west end. As with all camps in the devastated area, there is no shade and almost no protection from the wind.

The trail climbs steadily from Obscurity Lake to a narrow pass, and then descends toward deep Panhandle Lake. About halfway around the south shore of this scenic lake a downhill spur trail leads to the designated campsites near the lake's inlet creek.

Either Obscurity or Panhandle Lake is a fine place to spend the night, but don't stop your hike there. After setting up camp, take the time for a terrific side trip along the Lakes Trail to the west. The trail, which steeply ascends a ridge, offers some incredibly dramatic views down into the deep cirque of Shovel Lake. The tall, snow-streaked cliffs of Mt. Whittier rise above the cirque, making for dramatic photographs. As you gain elevation, you also gain increasingly excellent views of Mt. Adams to the east and Mt. Rainier and the Green River Valley to the north. You might also be fortunate enough to see the herd of elk that spends its summers in the high meadows of this region. At a ridgetop junction about

1 mile from Panhandle Lake a spur trail goes left and drops steeply to the west end of Shovel Lake where there are a couple of designated campsites. The main trail continues straight from this junction, contouring for 0.5 mile to a wide pass and a junction with the Whittier Ridge Trail.

NOTE

The map shows an enticing loop possibility that goes southeast on the Whittier Ridge Trail to a junction with the Boundary Trail. A hiker could then turn east and walk back to Bear Pass to close out the loop. Unfortunately, the Whittier Ridge Trail is so rugged, faint, and dangerously steep, it should only be contemplated by daring and athletic hikers with no fear of heights.

It is especially dangerous if snow remains on the trail or if rockslides and landslides have obliterated the narrow path (something that happens almost every year). It is safer and usually better to simply return the way you came.

15 Lewis River Trail

RATINGS	Scenery **5** Difficulty **2** Solitude **6**
ROUND-TRIP DISTANCE	5.2 miles (or more depending on your ambitions)
ELEVATION GAIN	200 feet
OPTIONAL MAP	*Green Trails: Lone Butte*
USUALLY OPEN	April to November
BEST TIMES	Mid-April to mid-October
AGENCY	Mount St. Helens National Volcanic Monument (Gifford Pinchot National Forest)
PERMIT	None

Highlights

Draining off the snowfields of Mt. Adams, the clear-flowing Lewis River cascades along through some of the most impressive forests and wooded canyons of our region. A trail once followed this magnificent stream all the way from the farmlands in the lower valley to the alpine terrain of the high country, but logging roads have long since destroyed virtually all of it. A much shortened, but still very worthwhile segment remains, however, and it is a joy to hike, with great camps, a fine swimming hole, good fishing, and some of the most impressive big trees in our region.

Getting There

Leave Interstate 5 north of Vancouver, Washington, at Woodland Exit 21 and travel 23.5 miles east on Highway 503 to a junction. Go straight on Highway 503 Spur and proceed 24.2 miles to a junction immediately past the Pine Creek Information Station. Turn right on paved Forest Road 90, drive 5.2 miles, and then turn sharply left on

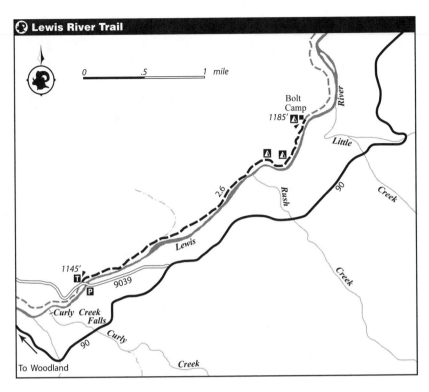

gravel Curly Creek Road (Road 9039). Proceed 0.7 mile to the signed trailhead immediately after a bridge over Lewis River.

Hiking It

Head upstream on a trail that parallels the north bank of the beautifully clear and rushing Lewis River. As pretty as the water is, rivaling the stream for your attention are the trees. Huge old Douglas firs and western red cedars mix with western hemlocks and moss-draped bigleaf maples, vine maples, and red alders in a grand display that resembles a living cathedral. Beneath this green canopy is a dense understory of salal, Oregon grape, sword fern, maidenhair fern, and various mosses and forest wildflowers. With all this

awe-inspiring old-growth, "grand" is hardly an adequate adjective to describe this forest, but it will have to do until the English language comes up with something better.

After just a few yards there is a fork in the trail. The 25-yard downhill path to the right provides quick access to the river, but the main trail keeps left on the hillside above the water. Like most river trails, this wide route includes several small ups and downs, but it is generally a long, gradual uphill either on the hillside a little above the river or on heavily forested, river-level flats. There are also several places where you can visit the water, do a little fishing, let the kids splash around, or just sit back and be soothed by the sounds of a flowing stream.

At 2.3 miles you pass a nice campsite just past where Rush Creek enters on the other side of the river. About 100 yards later is an even better campsite, this one right beside a superb swimming hole complete with a rope swing so you can do your best Tarzan imitation before plunging into the deep water. It is hard to imagine a more pleasant and enjoyable spot for a family backpacking trip.

Just 0.3 mile past this campsite is Bolt Camp, which has several fine tent sites clustered around a broken-down wooden shelter. The shelter looks like it will collapse the next time somebody sneezes, so it is probably safer to set up camp on the flat ground away from the structure.

Stronger hikers who want a bit more exercise can continue upstream on the Lewis River Trail another 6.7 miles, passing through fine forests and enjoying continuously attractive riverside scenes the entire distance. A particularly noteworthy highlight comes at just over 7 miles from the trailhead

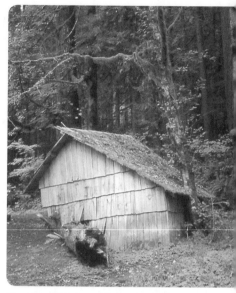

Dilapidated Bolt Camp Shelter, Lewis River Trail

when you climb to a fine clifftop viewpoint above the river. By making a short car shuttle you can turn this into a fun point-to-point 9.3-mile hike that exits at an upper trailhead on Road 90.

16 Quartz Creek

RATINGS	Scenery **5**　Difficulty **3**　Solitude **8**
ROUND-TRIP DISTANCE	9.2 miles
ELEVATION GAIN	750 feet
OPTIONAL MAP	*Green Trails: Lone Butte*
USUALLY OPEN	April to November
BEST TIMES	June to mid-October
AGENCY	Mount St. Helens National Volcanic Monument (Gifford Pinchot National Forest)
PERMIT	None

Highlights

Quartz Creek is that most precious of rarities in our region, a significant lower-elevation watershed that has largely

escaped the ravages of the chainsaw. Although there are a few logging scars in the creek's lower reaches, the generally undisturbed condition of the watershed ensures that the stream runs beautifully clear and cold beneath a green canopy of old-growth trees. That alone would make a visit here worthwhile, but the creek also has waterfalls, wildlife, and plenty of solitude, so despite the lack of distant views, hiking here is a joy.

Getting There

Leave Interstate 5 north of Vancouver, Washington, at Woodland Exit 21 and travel 23.5 miles east on Highway 503 to a junction. Go straight on Highway 503 Spur and proceed 24.2 miles to a junction immediately past the Pine Creek Information Station. Turn right on paved Forest Road 90 and drive 17 miles to a trailhead pullout just before a bridge over Quartz Creek.

Hiking It

The trail goes upstream on the west side of clear-flowing Quartz Creek

through a lush, old-growth forest of massive Douglas firs, western hemlocks, and western red cedars. After just 60 yards go straight at an unsigned junction with a spur trail that goes left to a horse camp. The trail then closely follows the creek for 0.4 mile before crossing Platinum Creek and making two uphill switchbacks that mark the beginning of a series of steep ups and downs. Although this part of the hike takes you well away from the creek, it compensates you with good, if partially obstructed, views of the creek canyon and surrounding ridges.

At 2 miles the trail descends to a crossing of Straight Creek. In late summer this is a simple rock-hop crossing, but early in the season it can be a wet and treacherous ford. There is a spacious and comfortable campsite on the north side of this crossing. Just downstream from this campsite, at the confluence of Straight and Quartz

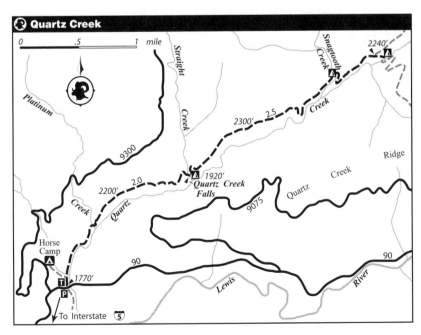

creeks, is 20-foot-tall Quartz Creek Falls, which drops into an inviting (but frigid!) swimming hole.

Past Straight Creek the trail makes a short, fairly steep climb, and then skirts the edge of a recovering clearcut before gradually descending once again to Quartz Creek. You continue upstream to a rock-hop crossing of Snagtooth Creek at 4.1 miles, and, 150 yards later, pass a mediocre campsite. To reach the best overnight spot in the canyon, continue another 0.4 mile to a fork, bear right (downhill), and walk 0.1 mile to an inviting campsite just before a chilly ford of Quartz Creek. This is the perfect place to spend the night admiring big trees while being serenaded by the soothing "river music" of a forest stream.

17 Siouxon Creek

RATINGS	Scenery **7** Difficulty **2** Solitude **4**
ROUND-TRIP DISTANCE	7.6 miles
ELEVATION GAIN	700 feet
OPTIONAL MAP	*Green Trails: Lookout Mountain*
USUALLY OPEN	March to November
BEST TIMES	May to October
AGENCY	Mount St. Helens National Volcanic Monument (Gifford Pinchot National Forest)
PERMIT	None

Highlights

Three of the trademark features of the Pacific Northwest—big trees, clear creeks, and lovely waterfalls—are all on spectacular display along Siouxon Creek. Flowing through an almost unlogged low-elevation valley, Siouxon Creek runs clear and cold, just the way a natural stream should flow in this part of the world. When combined with the majestic old-growth forest and several stunning waterfalls, this trip makes for a great introduction to the Northwest outdoors. The trail is very popular with mountain bikers, so hikers should expect to meet some cyclists along the way.

Getting There

From the intersection of State Highways 502 and 503 in downtown Battleground, Washington, drive 16.8 miles north on Highway 503 to a junction just after you pass the Mount St. Helens National Volcanic Monument Headquarters. Turn right on N.E. Healy Road and drive 9.2 miles to a poorly signed junction, where you bear left onto single-lane, paved Forest Road 57. Drive another 1.3 miles, and then turn sharply left on Forest Road 5701. Follow this rough, paved road for 3.7 miles to its end at a trailhead parking lot.

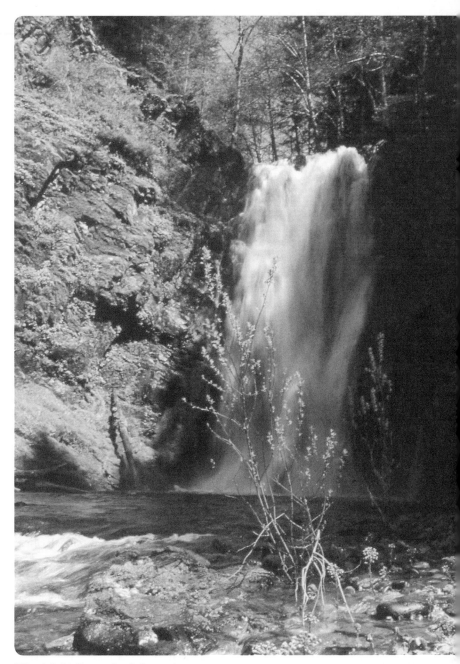

Chinook Falls, Siouxon Creek Area

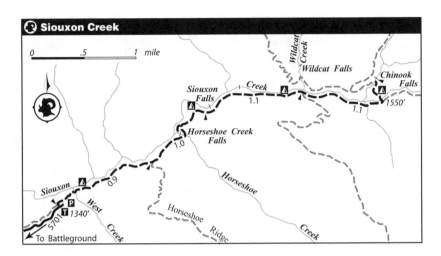

Hiking It

The trail departs from the north side of the lot and drops 50 feet to a junction with the Siouxon Creek Trail. Turn right and descend through a lovely forest composed predominantly of western hemlocks. On the forest floor are downed "nurse" logs sprouting a new growth of mosses, sword ferns, oxalis, and young saplings. After 0.1 mile of downhill, you reach and cross West Creek on a flat-topped log bridge. The walls of this creek's lush canyon are draped with mosses and ferns. Immediately after the bridge, you pass the first of this trip's many excellent campsites along clear Siouxon Creek. Although it occasionally approaches the water, the trail generally travels in small ups and downs staying about 50 feet above Siouxon Creek. At 0.9 mile is the signed junction with the Horseshoe Ridge Trail.

The Siouxon Creek Trail goes straight and does a series of small ups and downs, alternating between creek-level flats covered with a tangle of vegetation and hillsides sprouting

tall cedars, firs, and hemlocks. Several tiny tributary creeks cross the trail, providing ample water for plants such as devil's club and salmonberry. Cross Horseshoe Creek on a plank bridge just above lacy Horseshoe Creek Falls and, about 100 yards later, come to a junction with a 0.1-mile spur trail to a viewpoint at the base of this impressive falls.

About 0.2 mile after Horseshoe Creek Falls is a camp with a little wooden bench where you can sit and enjoy a classic view of nearby Siouxon Falls, a twisting cataract with a deep swimming hole at its base.

WARNING

The scramble down to this swimming hole is steep and difficult, especially if conditions are wet.

A short distance farther upstream you come to a smaller waterfall, and then hike past a series of unsigned side trails that lead to terrific campsites and lunch spots that are perfect places for the kids to play or for adults to quietly contemplate nature.

At 3 miles you reach the unsigned junction with the upper end of the Horseshoe Ridge Trail, which bears uphill to the right. You stay straight on the lower path and walk 0.7 mile to a junction right next to a bridge. The official Siouxon Creek Trail continues straight, reaching Forest Road 58 in about 4.5 miles. A more attractive route turns left, crosses the bridge above a deep pool of water, and wanders through forest for less than 0.1 mile to a pair of excellent campsites. From here the trail follows Chinook Creek upstream about 0.2 mile to the base of Chinook Falls, a scenic 50-foot drop over a sheer cliff. This is a great place to enjoy the scenery while having a snack and watching the kids play in the water.

If you are up for a bit more exploring, cross Chinook Creek and make a short traverse across a hillside to a junction with the Chinook Trail. Turn left and travel gently downhill for 0.5 mile to a bridgeless but easy crossing of Wildcat Creek, a little above where this stream joins Siouxon Creek. Turn right at an unofficial junction and climb 0.2 mile to a viewpoint at the base of impressive 100-foot-tall Wildcat Falls. Having enjoyed your fill of trees, creeks, and waterfalls, return the way you came.

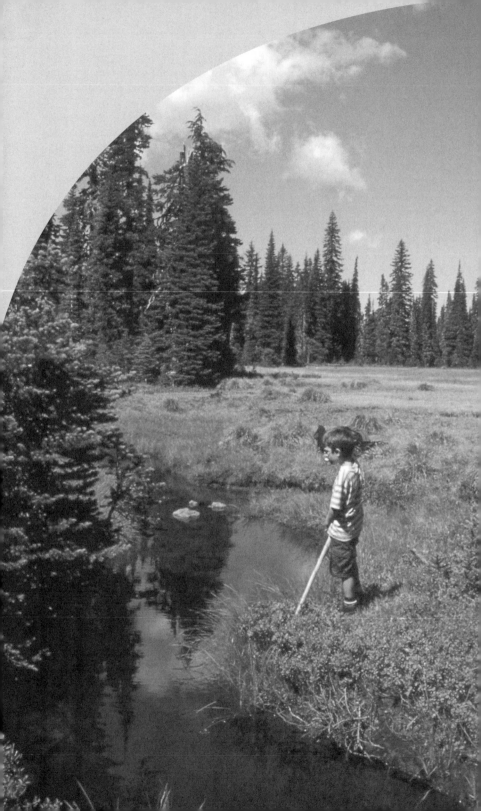

Mount Adams and Indian Heaven

Bulky Mt. Adams, which at 12,276 feet ranks second in our region only to Mt. Rainier in both its height and its girth, towers over the Cascade Range well to the east of most other major Cascade volcanoes. This easterly location means you have to drive a bit farther to reach the mountain, but also has some distinct advantages. First, the longer drive means that this peak, while just as scenic as its rivals, gets somewhat fewer visitors on its wildflower-covered slopes. Second, being farther east means that it is common, especially in the summer, for the clouds that frequently hang onto the western slopes of the Cascade Mountains to dissipate by the time they reach Mt. Adams, leaving this glacier-clad behemoth in brilliant sunshine. Not far to the southeast of Mt. Adams is a somewhat less dramatic but equally beautiful area called Indian Heaven. This gentle landscape hides hundreds of small lakes, open forests, and stunningly beautiful meadows. The wilderness here is especially attractive in early October, when the vine maples and huckleberry bushes turn red and orange, putting on one of the finest fall-color displays in the Pacific Northwest.

18 Dark Meadow via Jumbo Peak

RATINGS	Scenery **8** Difficulty **8** Solitude **8**
ROUND-TRIP DISTANCE	14 miles; 15.8 miles with side trip to Sunrise Peak
ELEVATION GAIN	3100 feet; 4000 feet with side trip to Sunrise Peak
OPTIONAL MAPS	*Green Trails: Blue Lake, McCoy Peak*
USUALLY OPEN	Late June to October
BEST TIMES	Early to mid-July
AGENCY	Cowlitz Valley Ranger District (Gifford Pinchot National Forest)
PERMIT	None

Highlights

If you like ridge walks through acres of wildflowers, past scenic rock formations, and to great viewpoints, then this is the trail for you. The Juniper Ridge Trail traces the entire length of its 13-mile-long, north-south-oriented namesake ridge, and hiking the entire distance is one of the finest ridge walks in our region. Since the full trail is more than most people want to tackle in a weekend, you might prefer this shorter version that hits most of the best sections, including the most interesting rock outcroppings and some of the best viewpoints. Although various species of wildflowers are abundant throughout, the real star of the show is beargrass, which in early to mid-July of favorable years puts on an amazing show of millions of tall stalks with clusters of tiny white blossoms.

The entire length of this trail is open to motorcycles. These infernal machines are not only noisy and annoying, they leave behind very badly eroded trails. Until this area is protected from the accursed machines, as wilderness or by some other designation, the abuses of these two-wheeled terrors will continue. One way to avoid these menaces is to hike early in the season before the trail maintenance has been completed. A few downed logs will usually keep out the motorcycles, while hikers can just crawl over the obstacles.

Getting There

Leave Interstate 5 north of Vancouver, Washington, at Exit 68 and drive east on U.S. Highway 12 for 48 miles to a junction at Randle. Turn right (south) on State Highway 131, following signs to Mt. St. Helens, and go 1 mile to a junction. Turn left onto Forest Road 23 and stay on this good paved road for 18.1 miles, past several intersections, to a major junction. Bear right, still on Road 23, which is now a winding one-lane road, proceed 4.6 miles, and then veer right onto gravel Road 2324, following signs to Surprise Peak Trail. Drive this steep, narrow, and sometimes rough road for 5.4 miles, fork left (uphill) at a junction, and continue a final 0.3 mile to the road-end turnaround and trailhead.

Hiking It

From the trailhead you can see your first goal, pointed Sunrise Peak, rising

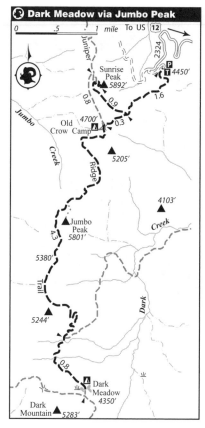

Dark Meadow via Jumbo Peak

0   .5   1   mile   To US 12

Juniper

Sunrise
Peak
5892'

P
4450'

2324

1.6

0.8   0.9

Old   4700'
Crow Camp   0.3

Jumbo
Creek

Ridge

5205'

4103'

Jumbo
Peak   Creek
5801'

4.3

5380'

Trail

5244'

Dark

0.8

Dark
Meadow
4350'

Dark
Mountain   5283'

Washington, Mounts Rainier, Adams, and St. Helens. In the distance to the south you can also see horn-shaped Mt. Hood in Oregon.

Back on the main trail, you descend across grassy slopes for 0.3 mile to an open saddle and a junction with the Juniper Ridge Trail. Turn left and, 100 yards later, meet an unmarked boot path that leads right 0.1 mile to Old Crow Camp. This is a scenic location in a lovely green basin, but the only water comes from snowmelt or a tiny, unreliable creek. The trail now climbs a series of open slopes north of prominent Jumbo Peak. Fires swept over this ridge in the early 1900s and the forests have yet to recover. As a result there are frequent excellent views and plenty of sunshine for colorful July-blooming wildflowers. Look for lupine, larkspur, paintbrush, wallflower, lomatium, cat's ear, yarrow, tiger lily, and phlox, among others. You can also expect to see hummingbirds, seemingly hundreds of which are attracted to the colorful, nectar-bearing flowers. The best views are looking north to Sunrise Peak, Mt. Rainier, and the Goat Rocks.

After making an irregular but very scenic climb, you reach the northern base of Jumbo Peak. The easiest way to reach the top of this cliff-edged high point is to scramble up the trailless north ridge. The views are well worth the extra sweat. The main trail loops around the towering cliffs on the west side of Jumbo Peak, and then comes to an open ridge south of the peak.

From the high, open slopes around Jumbo Peak the trail goes down along the ridge, and then steeply descends to the east. Initially you travel through a dense forest where snow often blocks the trail in early summer, but then you leave the forest and switchback down open slopes. Go left (downhill) at an

on the ridge to the west. To reach it, the trail winds up a side ridge partly in forest, but mostly across open, southeast-facing slopes with good views and plenty of wildflowers. At 1.6 miles is a junction. An excellent and highly recommended side trip goes to the right and makes a moderately steep climb for 0.6 mile up the mostly open southwest side of Sunrise Peak to a junction. From there you turn right and switchback uphill another 0.3 mile to the top of Sunrise Peak. A metal handrail helps to steady you on the final, rocky 50 feet. Views from here include all the nearby ridges and valleys, as well as the three major volcanic peaks of southern

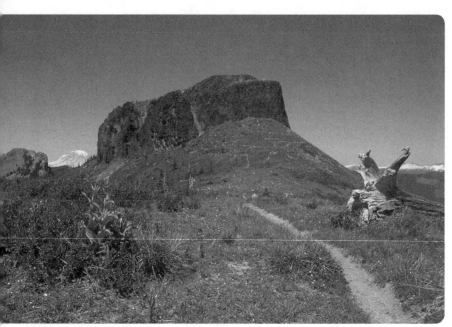

Jumbo Peak

unmarked junction with a long-abandoned trail and continue to a junction with little-used Dark Meadows Trail #263. Here you go straight and travel through brush and open forest, crossing several seasonal creeks on the way to misnamed Dark Meadow. This two-tiered, emerald-green gem sits beneath the cliffs and brushy slopes of Dark Mountain and is a good place to enjoy the wildflowers and watch for elk. The animals often spend their evenings here enjoying the pleasant diversions of bugling at one another and wallowing

in the mud. There are some nice camps beside the meadow and plenty of water, at least until about late July. You should expect mosquitoes in this marshy environment in early summer. Just beyond the camps the trail goes through an open forest between the two levels of Dark Meadow, before arriving at a T junction with the Boundary Trail. This motorcycle-plagued pathway leads to many fine destinations, but these are beyond the scope of a short backpacking trip.

19 Foggy Flat and Avalanche Valley

RATINGS	Scenery **10** Difficulty **10** Solitude **5**
ROUND-TRIP DISTANCE	13.5 miles to Foggy Flat; 24.4 miles to Avalanche Valley
ELEVATION GAIN	1300 feet to Foggy Flat; 4800 feet to Avalanche Valley
OPTIONAL MAP	*Green Trails: Mount Adams*
USUALLY OPEN	Late July to early October
BEST TIMES	August to early September
AGENCY	Mount Adams Ranger District (Gifford Pinchot National Forest) and Yakama Nation
PERMIT	Required. Forest Service permits are free at the trailhead. Hikers are technically supposed to obtain a permit for entry onto the Yakama Reservation around Avalanche Valley, but there is no reasonable way to do this, so the Yakamas do not currently enforce this requirement.

to Foggy Flat

Highlights

Avalanche Valley is one of that handful of indescribably spectacular places that every Northwest backpacker should visit at least once in their hiking lives. The joyful springs, lovely ponds, acres of wildflowers, and, most of all, amazing views of the massive east face of Mt. Adams make this one of our region's most outstanding backcountry locations. Getting there involves a long and fairly difficult hike, but almost every hiker who has made the effort swears that it is worth it.

Getting There

Drive 60 miles east of Portland on Interstate 84 to Hood River, take Exit 64, and cross the toll bridge into Washington ($.75 as of 2008). Turn left (west) on State Highway 14, drive 1.6 miles to a junction, then turn right (north) on Highway 141 ALT. Proceed 2.2 miles, turn left on Highway 141, and go 19.5 miles to a junction just before you enter the small town of Trout Lake. Turn right (north), following signs to Mt. Adams

Recreation Area, and drive 1.3 miles to a fork. Bear left onto Road 23 and remain on this paved then good gravel road through several intersections for 24 miles to a prominent junction. Turn right on Forest Road 2329 and follow this paved route to Takhlakh Lake. Drive past the campground at this popular lake and follow the narrow gravel road as it winds through forest and past trailheads for 9.5 miles to a junction with paved Road 5603. Turn right and drive 1.5 miles to the well-marked PCT Trailhead.

Hiking It

Walk south on the wide Pacific Crest Trail (PCT) as it gradually climbs through a lodgepole-pine forest for 1.9 miles to a large lava flow. The trail then rounds the end of this jumbled mass of dark rock and comes to cheerful little Lava Spring, where there is a fine campsite. After following the edge of the lava flow for another 0.5 mile, the trail angles away from the rock and goes briefly through forest to a bridged crossing of Muddy Fork Cispus River, a torrent of silt-laden glacial water. Just 0.1 mile later you cross a clear but unnamed creek, which has a good campsite on its south bank.

At 4.3 miles is a four-way junction with the Muddy Meadows Trail. Turn left and ascend through generally viewless forest for 1.9 miles before passing a nice campsite and coming to a junction with Highline Trail. Turn left and make a series of steep little ups and downs (more ups than downs) before coming to a lush, flat meadow called Foggy Flat. A clear stream flows through this green oasis, and there are excellent camps in the nearby forest. To the south, Mt. Adams picturesquely crowns the entire scene. As always, do not camp on the fragile meadow vegetation. Since the creek at Foggy Flat is the last good source of clear water for several miles, it is important that hikers fill their water bottles here.

The Yakama Nation no longer allows overnight camping in Avalanche Valley, so Foggy Flat is the last good, legal camping area on this trip. The best plan is to set up your tent, get a good night's sleep, and then begin early the next morning on the long but very rewarding dayhike into Avalanche Valley.

Beyond Foggy Flat the trail soon leaves the forest and enters a rugged area of boulders and glacial outwash. At the edge of this wasteland is a mediocre but acceptable camp near a small, reasonably clear creek. As the trail continues uphill the views, especially to the north of distant Mt. Rainier and the Goat Rocks, become ever more impressive. Another consequence of the increase in elevation is a change in the vegetation. The dense forest of earlier in the trip is replaced by just a few weather-stunted mountain hemlocks

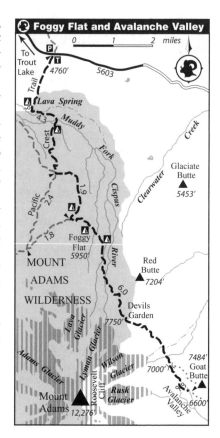

and whitebark pines. Even grass is rare in this rocky and inhospitable environment. The only animals you are likely to see are marmots and pikas, along with the occasional raven flying overhead. The path climbs steeply beside the upper reaches of Muddy Fork Cispus River, a boisterous glacial stream, and then drops briefly to cross the creek. Snowbridges provide reasonably safe passage across the torrent for most of the summer, but you should probe carefully with an ice ax or a walking stick to avoid thin spots. If the snowbridge has collapsed, the crossing may be very difficult or even dangerous. Have a rope on hand to assist weaker members of your group across. After crossing the creek, look for huge rock cairns on the far side and follow these as the trail resumes climbing through this above-timberline moonscape.

You climb moderately steeply through more boulder fields and lava, and then reach a small flat area covered with volcanic cinders. Here you will enjoy fine views of Red Butte, a prominent cinder cone about 1 mile to the northeast, and the distant icy summit of Mt. Rainier. The trail finally tops out at about 7750 feet on an exposed ridge called Devils Garden. Winds are almost constant here, so you may have to take cover behind one of the large rock cairns to rest and enjoy the view. Do not attempt this exposed section in bad weather.

The route now turns east and enters the Yakama Reservation. Beyond this point the trail exists only by virtue of hikers' boots, as the Yakamas do not maintain this remote route. In places the trail is sketchy and rough, but experienced hikers should have no difficulty. To ensure that the Yakama tribe is not forced to impose restrictions on public use, it is important that you never build fires and always treat the land with special care.

The scenic tour goes east to a small drop-off and then descends steeply over a semipermanent snowfield into a little basin. From here you turn south and cross rolling alpine terrain that is both varied and attractive, with many large boulders, pretty meadows, small creeks, and rocky ridges. Unfortunately, water sources in this sandy, volcanic soil sometimes dry up by late summer, so come prepared for a dry walk. Since the trail is easy to lose in this open

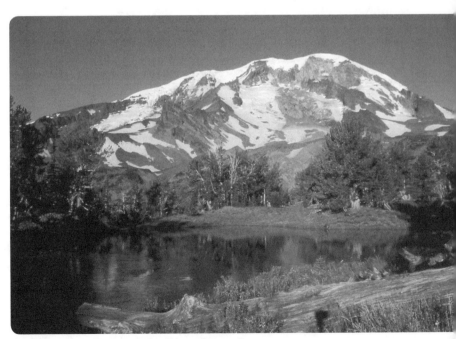

Mount Adams over Avalanche Valley, Yakama Reservation

terrain, you will need to watch carefully for small cairns that hikers have put up to aid in navigation.

The trail gradually descends to cross a couple of usually flowing creeks draining out of Wilson Glacier, and then climbs a little to a low saddle northwest of prominent Goat Butte. From this saddle the trail descends past some springs to two small but very scenic ponds before dropping to the glorious expanse of Avalanche Valley. A large, gushing spring gives birth to a good-sized creek of *extremely* cold water at the head of the meadows, while colorful wildflowers carpet the area. The craggy edge of Goat Butte forms a beautiful backdrop along the meadow's eastern edge. It will be hard to notice any of these features, however, as your attention will naturally be turned to the jaw-dropping view of Mt. Adams to the west. Cliffs and 4000-foot-high ramparts support streaking waterfalls that pour out of Rusk and Klickitat glaciers, shimmering in the sun. Higher still rises Roosevelt Cliff, then more glaciers, and finally the rounded summit of the great volcano. The scene is truly outstanding and well worth several hours of gazing to appreciate. With binoculars you may even be able to pick out mountain goats on the cliffs.

If you have time for some exploring, go back up to the trail saddle northwest of Avalanche Valley, then climb southeast along a ridge to the summit of Goat Butte. The view from here of Mt. Adams to the west and the semi-desert of central Washington to the east is about as good as views get.

20 High Camp and Killen Creek

RATINGS	Scenery **9** Difficulty **6** Solitude **4**
ROUND-TRIP DISTANCE	8.2 miles to High Camp; 8.4 miles to Killen Creek; 10.4 miles combined
ELEVATION GAIN	2350 feet to High Camp; 1800 feet to Killen Creek; 2650 feet combined
OPTIONAL MAP	*Green Trails*: Mount Adams
USUALLY OPEN	Mid-July to October
BEST TIMES	Late July through August
AGENCY	Mount Adams Ranger District (Gifford Pinchot National Forest)
PERMIT	Required. Free at the trailhead.

to Killen Creek

Highlights

Aptly named High Camp sits at timberline on the northwest shoulder of Mt. Adams, and, like most such high-elevation locations, it offers views that are absolutely stupendous. Most impressive are those looking up to the hulking mass of the nearby mountain, but you can also enjoy distant views to other volcanic peaks, including Mt. Hood, Mt. Rainier, and Mt. St. Helens, and look across thousands of square miles of forested ridges and valleys. The sunsets from this camp are frequently breathtaking. But like most timberline locations, High Camp is very exposed to the weather. Winds are nearly constant (good for keeping bugs at bay, but bad for almost everything else), and if a storm is on the way, it can be mighty uncomfortable. For an alternate destination a bit lower on the mountain, try Killen Creek, which has lesser views, but provides more comfortable camping. Here you will find an often crowded but nice camp amid a protective grove of trees, a delightful waterfall, and a pretty little pond with a superb reflection of Mt. Adams. The two locations are close enough to be combined in a single hike, but are worth enjoying separately on different trips.

Getting There

Drive 60 miles east of Portland on Interstate 84 to Hood River, take Exit 64, and cross the toll bridge into Washington ($.75 as of 2008). Turn left (west) on State Highway 14, drive 1.6 miles to a junction, then turn right (north) on Highway 141 ALT. Proceed 2.2 miles, turn left on Highway 141, and go 19.5 miles to a junction just before you enter the small town of Trout Lake. Turn right (north), following signs to Mt. Adams Recreation Area, and drive 1.3 miles to a fork. Bear left onto Road 23 and remain on this paved then good gravel road through several intersections for 24 miles to a prominent junction. Turn right on Forest Road 2329 and follow this paved route to a junction with the entrance road to popular Takhlakh Lake Campground. Go straight, follow the narrow gravel road for 4.4 miles, and then turn right into the Killen Creek Trailhead.

Hiking It

The trail winds its way south, initially on an old jeep road, but then following a pleasant trail through a forest of lodgepole pines and other conifers with a dense understory dominated by beargrass and tall huckleberry bushes. The steadily uphill route is mostly in viewless forest, but with plenty of small wildflowers and an unusual variety of mushrooms along the way to keep your interest. Unfortunately, the trail is often very dusty, due to rather heavy horse use and a thick layer of light gray ash dropped here by Mt. St. Helens.

At about 2.5 miles the terrain becomes much more interesting when you enter some large meadows with lots of wildflowers. As with most mountain

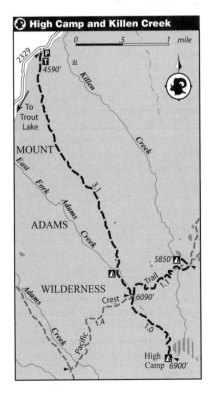

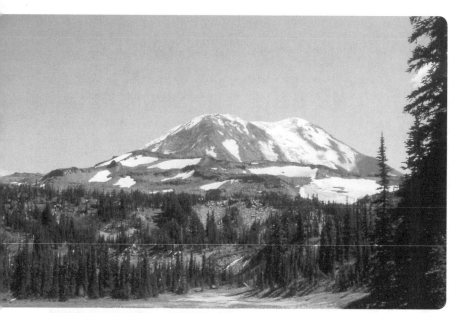

Mount Adams from Killen Creek Meadows

meadows, what is blooming depends on the season, with marsh marigold, shooting star, western anemone, and avalanche lily dominating in early summer; paintbrush, lupine, phlox, and pink heather taking over in midsummer; and gentian rounding out the show in late summer and early fall. The uphill in these meadows is more gradual than it was in the forest and is frequently interspersed with level stretches.

Shortly after passing a shallow, seasonal pond, the trail crosses tiny East Fork Adams Creek, which flows for most of the summer and has a nice campsite in a nearby grove of trees. A bit more uphill through meadows takes you to a four-way junction with the Pacific Crest Trail (PCT) at 3.1 miles.

If you are heading for High Camp, go straight at the junction and resume your uphill on a trail that takes you into increasingly rocky terrain. You are rapidly approaching timberline now, so what trees you find are mostly stunted whitebark pines. The trail skirts around a rocky cliff, and then passes a series of small meadows and semipermanent snowfields before making a final uphill push in short, rocky switchbacks to the small, mostly level plain holding High Camp. There are a few twisted pines here, but generally little else to provide shelter from the wind. Water is available either from seasonal snowmelt creeks or from lingering snow patches. Campfires are prohibited at this and any other site above the Pacific Crest Trail.

In good weather the explorations from High Camp are magnificent. There are no trails, but you can wander to your heart's content up rocky moraines, through alpine meadows, over old lava flows, and past small waterfalls. If you are really ambitious, you can even make your way up to the base of Adams Glacier. The views are outstanding, especially up to the rugged ramparts of Mt. Adams. Be sure to navigate carefully, however, because if the clouds move in, it can be very difficult to find your way back through this bleak, trailless terrain.

If you are visiting Killen Creek, return to the PCT junction and turn north on that well-traveled pathway as it winds its way up and down past meadows, over small ridges, and through bits of forest for almost 1 mile to a gorgeous meadow with a shallow little pond that is often fringed with thousands of tiny white flowers. Best of all, the pond features a fine view of

Mt. Adams. After rounding this small meadow you cross Killen Creek just above a beautiful sloping waterfall, descend a hillside just east of this falls, and come to a junction with an obvious spur trail that goes left to a nice but overused campsite in a grove of trees. This deservedly popular spot has a lovely setting just below the falls and access to a fairly large pond about 100 yards to the northwest with a superb view of Mt. Adams. Less crowded campsites are available if you hunt around in the forests and rocky areas to the west or by searching upstream along Killen Creek. As always, camp at least 100 feet from water.

21 Horseshoe Meadow and Crystal Lake

RATINGS	Scenery **7** Difficulty **6 to 8** Solitude **7**
ROUND-TRIP DISTANCE	14 miles to Horseshoe Meadow; 20 miles to Crystal Lake
ELEVATION GAIN	1400 feet to Horseshoe Meadow; 1900 feet to Crystal Lake
OPTIONAL MAP	*Green Trails: Mount Adams*
USUALLY OPEN	Mid-July to October
BEST TIMES	Late July to early October
AGENCY	Mount Adams Ranger District (Gifford Pinchot National Forest)
PERMIT	Required. Free at the trailhead. Northwest Forest Pass required.

Highlights

Although the Pacific Northwest has thousands of miles of trails leading to impressive and worthwhile locations, often the best and most beautiful spots are hidden just off the maintained paths. One such gem is Crystal Lake, on the southwest side of Mt. Adams. Although little more than a pond, the lake is perfectly situated to provide drop-dead gorgeous views of its neighboring glacier-clad peak. But since this

lake is not on an established trail, relatively few hikers make the detour to find and enjoy this spot. An alternate destination for hikers with a little less time and energy is Horseshoe Meadow, which also features a tremendous view of the mountain and has better displays of wildflowers.

Getting There

Drive 60 miles east of Portland on Interstate 84 to Hood River, take Exit 64

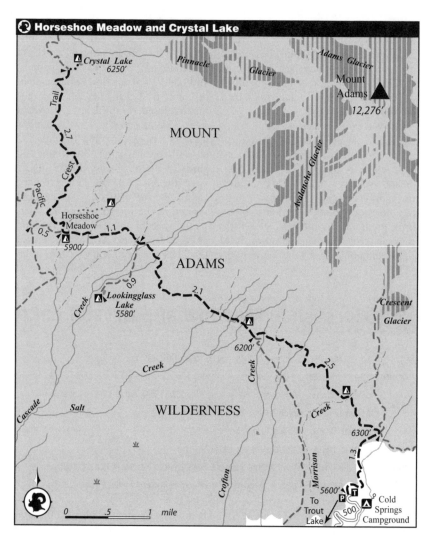

Horseshoe Meadow and Crystal Lake

and cross the toll bridge into Washington ($.75 as of 2008). Turn left (west) on State Highway 14, drive 1.6 miles to a junction, then turn right (north) on Highway 141 ALT. Proceed 2.2 miles, turn left on Highway 141, and go 19.5 miles to a junction just before you enter the small town of Trout Lake. Turn right (north), following signs to Mt. Adams Recreation Area, and drive 1.3 miles to a fork. Veer right and proceed 0.7 mile to another fork, where you go left onto Forest Road 80. Stay on this initially paved, then gravel road for about 9 miles to Morrison Creek Campground, where you turn right and continue 2.5 miles on rough dirt Road 500 to the trailhead near Cold Springs Campground. This trailhead parking area fills quickly with climbers looking to go up Mt. Adams, so try to arrive early.

Hiking It

Walk north on a wide trail (actually a long-abandoned jeep road) as you gradually gain elevation in an open forest of mountain hemlocks and subalpine firs. With each step the surroundings become increasingly alpine in nature, with more wildflowers and fewer trees. At 1.3 miles is a four-way junction with the Round-the-Mountain Trail. The well-used path that goes straight (uphill) is the most popular climbing route up Mt. Adams. The ascent is long and tiring, but not technically difficult. If you want to make the attempt, keep in mind that all climbers are required to have a Cascade Volcanoes Pass when venturing above 7000 feet on the mountain. As of 2008, daily passes cost $10 for a weekday or $15 for a weekend day and are available at the Mt. Adams Ranger Station in Trout Lake.

For this trip you turn left (west) at the junction and begin a long, gently rolling traverse that leads over a small ridge to a nice view of Mt. Adams. The terrain is generally open, with some mountain hemlocks adding patches of shade and variety. At 2.1 miles you cross intermittent Morrison Creek (adequate camps nearby), and then continue the easy up-and-down hike. On clear days this area provides some fine views looking south to Oregon's Mt. Hood. After crossing some old lava flows and a few usually dry creekbeds, you come to a junction with the Shorthorn Trail at 3.8 miles. Keep straight and soon reach Salt Creek, where there are some scenic camps.

The trail continues west, maintaining its remarkably level grade.

Although the trail is mostly gentle, the surrounding landscape is not, much of it consisting of jumbled rock and sand deposited here in a massive landslide in 1921. Another huge debris slide came down this side of Mt. Adams in 1997, although that one did not get as far down as the trail. In late 2006, several significant washouts occurred along this section when many of the creeks flooded and washed away the unstable soils. Be sure to check on current conditions before attempting this hike.

The trail eventually reenters gentler alpine terrain, and then crosses two branches of aptly named Cascade Creek just before reaching a junction. The trail to the left leads down to tiny Lookingglass Lake, which has some pleasant camps, but your trail goes straight and continues west for 1.1 miles to the welcome expanse of Horseshoe Meadow. This large and remarkably flat meadow is covered with tiny wildflowers in July and August and features an excellent view of Mt. Adams. The best views are from the southwest side of the meadow. The tiny creek crossing Horseshoe Meadow sometimes dries up by midsummer, but if water is available there are excellent camps near the creek crossing. Unfortunately, horse parties often use these camps, so expect plenty of horse "apples" and that distinctive equine aroma. For privacy and more reliable water, consider walking cross-country up to the northeast corner of the meadow, and then scrambling uphill past a waterfall on the right branch of the intermittent creek to a lovely pumice-covered meadow, where there are nice mountain views, good camps, and water from a permanent tributary of Cascade Creek.

At the west end of Horseshoe Meadow is a junction with the Pacific Crest

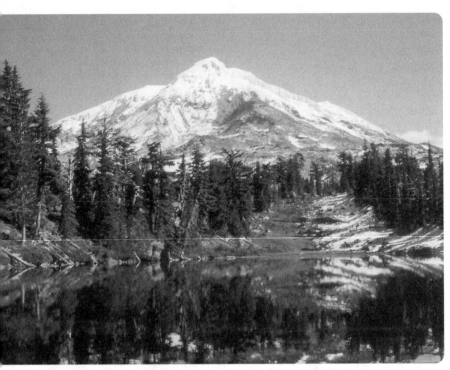

Mount Adams over Crystal Lake

Trail (PCT). Turn right (north), gain a little elevation along a minor ridge, and then make an up-and-down traverse of numerous small ridges and gullies on a circuitous course to the north. Views of Mt. Adams are blocked by ridges, but there are nice vistas to the west of distant Mt. St. Helens. You round a ridge, then about 2.7 miles from where you started on the PCT, you begin to lose elevation along the side of a second ridge. Immediately after beginning this descent, turn right (east) off the trail and walk cross-country up a grassy gully for 0.2 mile. From there you turn left and climb a rocky area with scattered trees to small Crystal Lake. The lake has no fish and is too cold for comfortable swimming, but the view of Mt. Adams across the glassy waters is superb. Be sure to camp at least 100 feet away from water in this pristine area.

22 Sunrise Camp

RATINGS	Scenery **9** Difficulty **8** Solitude **5**
ROUND-TRIP DISTANCE	8 miles
ELEVATION GAIN	2650 feet
OPTIONAL MAP	*Green Trails: Mount Adams* (but the trail alignment is inaccurate)
USUALLY OPEN	Late July to September
BEST TIMES	August and September
AGENCY	Yakama Nation
PERMIT	Yakama tribal permits are required both to enter and to camp in this area. Entry permits cost $5 per vehicle as of 2007 and can be purchased at the kiosk along the road near Mirror Lake. Camping permits cost $10 per group and can be purchased at the self-service drop box at the trailhead.

Highlights

Sunrise Camp, as the name suggests, is an excellent place to watch a sunrise, but there is much more to recommend this trip than just the fine early-morning show. Located high above timberline on the east slopes of Mt. Adams in the Yakama Indian Reservation, the camp is also a great place to observe mountain goats, take in extensive views, get up-close-and-personal with a glacier, and fill your lungs with clear mountain air. The hike, however, is not for everyone, as the upper part of the route involves boulder-hopping and off-trail scrambling. At least one member of the party should be familiar with cross-country travel. The camp is also very exposed, so bring a sturdy tent and do not attempt this hike in bad weather.

Getting There

Drive 60 miles east of Portland on Interstate 84 to Hood River, take Exit 64 and cross the toll bridge into Washington ($.75 as of 2008). Turn left (west) on State Highway 14, drive 1.6 miles to a junction, then turn right (north) on Highway 141 ALT. Proceed 2.2 miles, turn left on Highway 141, and go 19.5 miles to a junction just before you enter the small town of Trout Lake. Turn right (north), following signs to Mt. Adams Recreation Area, and drive 1.3 miles to a fork. Veer right on what becomes Forest Road 82 and drive 2.6 miles on this paved road to a multi-way junction at a Sno-Park, where the road turns to gravel. Continue on Road 82, following signs to Bird Creek Meadows, and proceed 6.4 miles on this good gravel road to another fork. Go straight on what quickly becomes a rough dirt road and slowly bounce along for 4.2 miles to a tribal pay station and road junction beside scenic little Mirror Lake. After buying your entry permit, go straight at the junction and drive 1.1 miles to the spacious trailhead parking area on the left.

Hiking It

The wide and often dusty trail (actually a long-abandoned road) goes west through a lovely high-elevation forest

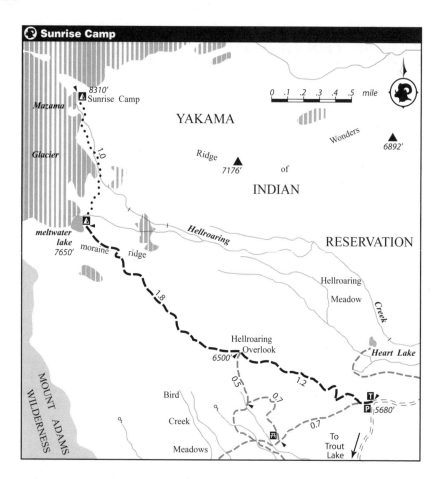

Sunrise Camp

of mountain hemlocks and subalpine firs, with a rather sparse understory of huckleberries, lupines, and various wildflowers. After only 0.1 mile you go right at a junction onto a foot trail signed as MOUNTAIN CLIMBERS TRAIL. This path winds uphill at an uneven but sometimes steep grade through a landscape that becomes increasingly open as you gain elevation. Initially, you catch only occasional glimpses of Mt. Adams, but these become more expansive and impressive as you continue uphill. The vegetation also changes to more alpine varieties, with wind-

twisted whitebark pines replacing the previous trees, and low-growing flowers such as late-August-blooming gentians becoming more dominant. At 1.2 miles you reach Hellroaring Overlook, where there is an outstanding view of the wide, steep-sided canyon of Hellroaring Creek and up to glacier-clad Mt. Adams. To the north you can see a tall waterfall dropping over the headwall of Hellroaring Canyon. Your route will take you a little above the top of this falls.

Above Hellroaring Overlook an unmaintained trail continues uphill, generally staying near the edge of the drop-off into Hellroaring Canyon. There are several unsigned use paths in this area, but if you stay close to the rim and stick with what appears to be the main route, it is hard to go wrong. If you lose the trail, look for occasional cairns or orange blazes on rocks to help get you back on track. As you continue gaining elevation the trees become smaller and then disappear entirely, leaving only rocks, grasses, small wildflowers, and plenty of amazing views. To the south you can see Mt. Hood and the high points of the Columbia River Gorge. To the east extend the forested Simcoe Mountains and the dry plains of eastern Washington. And, most impressive of all, straight ahead to the north rises huge Mt. Adams, covered with rocks, snow, and massive flows of ice. This is some of the best high country hiking in our region.

Since this trail is not maintained or signed and it travels through harsh and rocky terrain, you should expect to do some wandering around to find the correct route. This doesn't affect the scenery, but you need to realize that the mileages given here are only approximations. At about 2.7 miles you come to the top of a large moraine, left behind by the retreating Mazama Glacier. Turn left and go up the spine of this rocky moraine for about 100 yards, and then bear right on an obvious trail that makes a rough and rocky up-and-down traverse for 0.3 mile to a possible emergency campsite near a stark and unnamed meltwater lake at the base of Mazama Glacier. A few rocks have been piled around the tent site here to provide at least some shelter from the frequent winds. The lake is a spectacular spot, filled with floating icebergs for the two months each year it is not frozen over entirely. You can see a small part of the top of Mt. Adams over a ridge to the north.

Above the meltwater lake the way is only a general route. There is no tread visible amid the rocks, although a few cairns have been built to assist hikers with navigation. Fortunately, staying on course is surprisingly easy, as you simply make your way up toward the

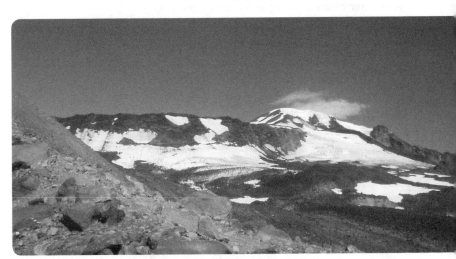

Mount Adams from moraine below Mazama Glacier, Yakama Reservation

left side of an obvious flat-topped ridge that extends east from the shoulder of Mt. Adams. The easiest route to this destination crosses the meltwater lake's silty outlet creek, and then climbs over rocks and snowfields going almost due north. You will cross a couple of very silty meltwater creeks along the way, but these crossings are easy rock-hops.

You reach the low point in the ridge at 4 miles, where you are greeted with a tumbling creek flowing from the icy base of nearby Mazama Glacier. Sunrise Camp is located on a large sandy flat with several tent sites. Once again campers have stacked up low rock walls to provide some protection from the almost constant winds. Even so, the area is very exposed, so you will need a sturdy tent with plenty of guy wires. If you can tear your eyes away from the amazing scenery, be sure to check the nearby rocky areas for mountain goats. Often the animals will wander right through camp, so guard your food carefully. Never approach the goats, which are unpredictable and possess very sharp horns.

It is possible to scramble from Sunrise Camp to Avalanche Valley (see Trip 19), which you can see well below you to the north-northeast. However, the way is unmarked, steep, rough, and potentially dangerous. Depending on conditions, you may have to cross glaciers and you will certainly have to negotiate steep rocky areas that are extremely difficult and even dangerous for novice hikers. It is better to return the way you came.

23 Lemei and Blue Lakes Loop

RATINGS	Scenery **7** Difficuly **4** Solitude **5**
ROUND-TRIP DISTANCE	12.3 miles (with many shorter options)
ELEVATION GAIN	1800 feet
OPTIONAL MAPS	*Green Trails: Lone Butte, Wind River* (although older trails are not shown)
USUALLY OPEN	Late June to October
BEST TIMES	Late August / early to mid-October
AGENCY	Mount Adams Ranger District (Gifford Pinchot National Forest)
PERMIT	Required. Free at the trailhead. Northwest Forest Pass required.

Highlights

The Indian Heaven Wilderness is a gentle mountain landscape that covers a high volcanic plateau in the Washington Cascades southwest of Mt. Adams. Instead of featuring a towering, glacier-clad mountain like many other wilderness areas in our region, this wilderness protects hundreds of lakes and beautiful subalpine meadows amid an open mid-elevation forest. Hiking here is relatively easy because elevation gains are generally small and there seems to be a new lake with fine campsites around every bend. Although in July the wildflowers are terrific, that is when the bugs in this area (sometimes called "Mosquito Heaven") can number in the trillions—and that's just counting the clouds hovering around your head. As a result, it is best to give this area a very wide berth in July and early August—a couple of hundred miles should do it. Fall-color time in early October is a much better time to visit, since the huckleberry bushes will be bright orange and red, the meadows golden brown, and the vine maples a stunning scarlet. Best of all, you probably won't see a single bug. Late August is also a good time for this trip, especially if you are a fan of eating tasty huckleberries.

NOTE

Although part of this loop is on abandoned trails that are no longer maintained or shown on the newer maps, they are still easy to follow and fun to hike.

Getting There

Drive Interstate 84 east to Cascade Locks, take Exit 44, and almost immediately veer right to loop around and cross the Columbia River on the Bridge of the Gods (a $1 toll applies, as of 2008). Turn right on State Highway 14, go 6.1 miles, and then turn left (north) on the signed road to Carson.

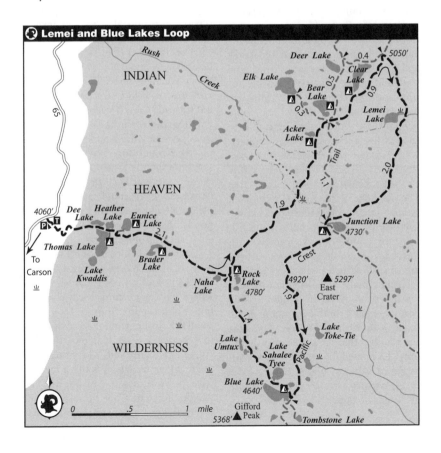

After 0.9 mile go straight at an intersection in the middle of Carson, and then proceed 4.9 miles to a junction. Turn right on Old State Road, proceed 0.1 mile, and then turn left on paved Forest Road 65. Follow this road for 11.1 miles to a four-way junction, where you go straight, still on paved Road 65. After 2 more miles you come to a fork where the pavement ends. Keep right on Road 65 and proceed a final 6.8 miles on good gravel to the signed Thomas Lake Trailhead on the right.

Hiking It

The trail starts in an old clear-cut, but soon leaves this unattractive area, enters the Indian Heaven Wilderness, and travels through a lovely mid-elevation forest of mountain hemlocks and Pacific silver firs. Tall blueberry and huckleberry bushes crowd the trail and make tempting reasons to stop and enjoy the harvest from late August to mid-September. The route is uphill, but never steep, and is easy enough for hikers of any age or ability. After 0.5 mile you reach the first lakes when the trail cuts through the narrow strip of forested land separating large Thomas Lake on the right (south) from smaller Dee and Heather lakes on the left (north). All three lakes have fish and are good for swimming. With such easy trail access, it is not surprising that these lakes are very popular. Still, they make excellent destinations for hikers with young children. The Forest Service prohibits camping in the fragile strip of land between the lakes and requires that backpackers only use sites designated by cedar posts with engraved camp symbols. Some of the best legal sites are along the east shore of Thomas Lake.

Near the southeast end of Heather Lake a spur trail goes straight 120 yards to a nice campsite beside pretty Eunice Lake. The main trail goes right at this junction, makes a very short but steep climb up a forested ridge, and then levels out as you enter the high plateau of Indian Heaven. This plateau is covered with forests and delightful meadows that are lined with low-growing huckleberries and heather. Unseen to the south is off-trail Brader Lake which you can wander down to and camp beside with a reasonable chance of privacy. The main trail continues straight, passing through more small meadows and strips of forest as it gradually climbs to an unsigned but obvious junction at 2.1 miles just 75 yards west of shallow Rock Lake.

The official trail goes sharply right (south) here, and is the way you will return if you take the recommended loop. For now, turn left on a section of the old Cascade Crest Trail and follow this winding and often badly eroded route as it goes downhill in fits and starts, mostly through forest for 0.7 mile before entering the large meadows in the center of Indian Heaven. These grassy expanses are stunningly attractive with plenty of wildflowers and several small ponds. In early to mid-October the color show is outstanding.

In the middle of one of these meadows the trail crosses a deep but sluggish section of misnamed Rush Creek, where kids can amuse themselves for hours hunting for frogs or looking at small fish. Just beyond this crossing you may notice a very faint old trail that angles off to the left. Go straight on the main route, which is often marked with posts across the meadows, and wander north to a fine campsite beside lovely Acker Lake. This lake is rarely

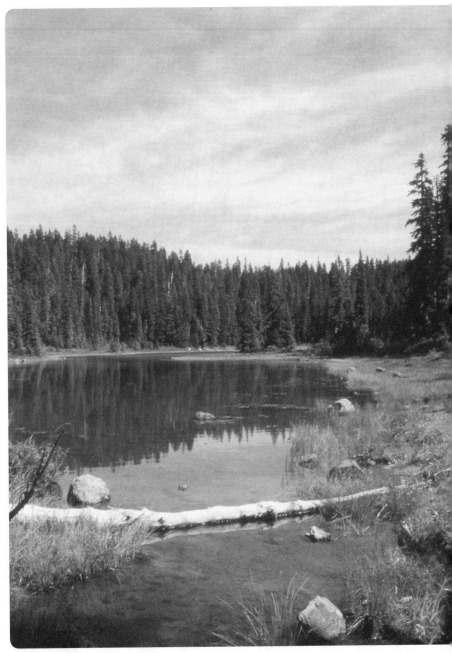

Junction Lake, Indian Heaven Wilderness

crowded, and makes a fine place to spend the night.

Beyond Acker Lake the old trail makes a short but steep climb up a forested hillside to a multiway junction. Through the trees to the north you can see deep Bear Lake. The main trail at this junction is the Pacific Crest Trail (PCT), which goes north and south. Another official trail goes left on its way to Elk Lake. Your route, however, goes straight across the PCT to the east, following another old trail that winds uphill beside a little gully. After about 0.2 mile look for a use path that continues upstream along the gully for about 50 yards to a fine campsite at the south end of large Clear Lake. This is a particularly beautiful lake, as its north end is backed by a scenic talus slope.

The main trail wanders up and down through the forests east of Clear Lake, eventually coming to a junction at 4.9 miles. Turn sharply right here onto the maintained Lemei Trail. This winding route takes you south through more meadow-and-forest country for 0.5 mile to the large meadow holding marshy Lemei Lake. This is an excellent place to eat lunch and enjoy the view to the east of distant Lemei Rock. The trail then makes a short uphill before heading southwest, mostly in forest, for another 1.5 miles to Junction Lake. This narrow lake features fine campsites and, true to its name, several trail junctions.

Turn south on the PCT, ignoring a junction with the East Lemei Trail that goes along the south side of Junction Lake, and climb a bit before making a long loop around the forested flanks of an old cinder cone called East Crater. At the south end of this traverse you lose elevation and then reach a junction at the eastern end of Blue Lake at 8.8 miles. Turn right at this junction,

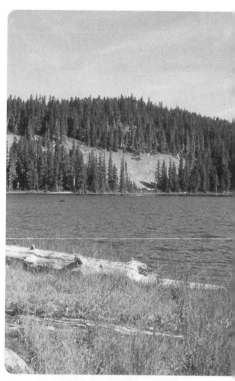

Clear Lake, Indian Heaven Wilderness

leaving the PCT, and soon pass some superb campsites above the northeast shore of the lake. This is a fairly popular but very scenic place to spend the night, because the deep, clear lake is backed by the impressive cliffs of Gifford Peak to the southwest. Backpackers are required to camp at sites designated by cedar posts with camp symbols.

To close out the loop, follow the trail as it goes uphill, rounds the shore of Lake Sahalee Tyee (more designated camps here), and then reenters meadow country as it winds past Lake Umtux and a series of nearby ponds back to the junction near Rock Lake. Turn left and return past Thomas Lake the way you came.

24 Lake Wapiki

RATINGS	Scenery **7** Difficulty **6** Solitude **6**
ROUND-TRIP DISTANCE	9.6 miles
ELEVATION GAIN	2500 feet
OPTIONAL MAPS	Green Trails: Lone Butte, Mount Adams—West
USUALLY OPEN	Late June to October
BEST TIMES	Late August / early October
AGENCY	Mount Adams Ranger District (Gifford Pinchot National Forest)
PERMIT	Required. Free at the trailhead. Northwest Forest Pass required.

Highlights

Filling the center of a colorful old volcanic crater, Lake Wapiki is one of the crown jewels in the string of watery gems that populate Washington's Indian Heaven Wilderness. There are two ways into the lake; the eastern approach is shorter and involves less elevation gain, but travels through viewless forest the entire way. The more attractive and recommended option comes in from the north and west on a very scenic route that visits lovely Cultus Lake, passes several beautiful meadows, takes you to a fine viewpoint, and nearly touches the jagged crags of dramatic Lemei Rock. Overall, it is a tasty package, and you can make it even tastier if you time your visit for late August when the huckleberries are ripe. As with other trips in Indian Heaven, avoid July and early August when you will be plagued by clouds of buzzing, blood-sucking mosquitoes.

Getting There

Drive 60 miles east of Portland on Interstate 84 to Hood River, take Exit 64, and cross the toll bridge into Washington ($0.75 as of 2007). Turn left (west) on State Highway 14, drive 1.6 miles to a junction, and then turn right (north) on Highway 141 ALT. Proceed 2.2 miles, turn left on Highway 141, and go 19.6 miles to the small town of Trout Lake. Stay on the main road through town, and then continue 8 miles to a junction. Paved Forest Road 60 goes straight, but turn right on good gravel Road 24 and continue for 9.1 miles to Cultus Creek Campground. Turn left and follow the dirt campground loop road for 0.2 mile to the signed trailhead.

Hiking It

Walk southwest from the campground through a dense but attractive forest of mixed conifers featuring grand firs, Douglas firs, Engelmann spruces, and western hemlocks. The forest floor is covered with a thick blanket of beargrass, vanilla leaf, and false hellebore, but the most common understory species here, as it is throughout Indian Heaven, is huckleberries. After crossing a trickling creek, the trail begins going uphill moderately steep. At 1.4 miles you briefly break out of the trees for a fine view of Mounts Adams and

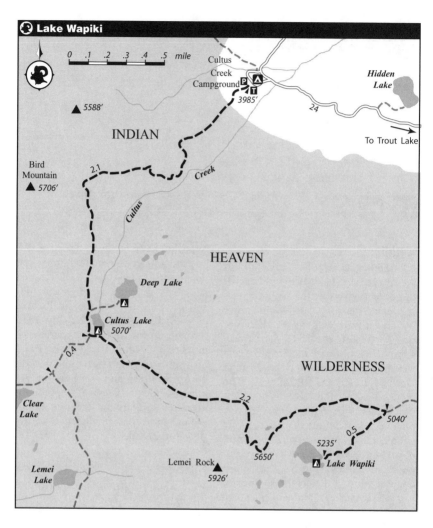

Rainier, and then return to forest and continue uphill, although now at a more gradual grade.

The terrain opens up at 1.5 miles, where the forest is interspersed with delightful subalpine meadows filled with grasses, wildflowers, and low-growing huckleberry bushes. In early October these bushes turn bright orange and red, making for a great display of color. In addition to being beautiful, these meadows provide fine views of nearby rugged peaks such as Bird Mountain and Lemei Rock.

At 2 miles you reach Cultus Lake and a signed junction with the short side trail to aptly named Deep Lake, which features a nice view of distant Mt. Adams. Huckleberry bushes line the shores of both Deep and Cultus lakes, as they do all area meadows and bodies of water in this wilderness.

Above the southwest end of Cultus Lake are a very good campsite and a trail junction. To reach Lake Wapiki, turn left on the Lemei Trail, which for the next mile or so climbs through stunningly beautiful meadows that come alive in late July with the blossoms of pink heather, white partridgefoot, blue lupine, and numerous other colorful wildflowers. At 3.4 miles the trail tops a ridge that radiates off the northeast shoulder of jagged Lemei Rock. From here you turn left to cross a small open area with outstanding views down into the deep bowl holding Lake Wapiki and northeast to snow-covered Mt. Adams.

The trail now makes a rather steep descent, losing 600 feet in 0.9 mile, to a signed junction with a 0.5-mile uphill spur trail leading to the east end of Lake Wapiki. There are several fine campsites at this very scenic lake, which allow you to put up your tent and spend a lazy afternoon fishing or just gazing in admiration at the lake and its surrounding ridges. Since this is one of our area's best swimming lakes, you will probably want to plunge in and give that a try as well.

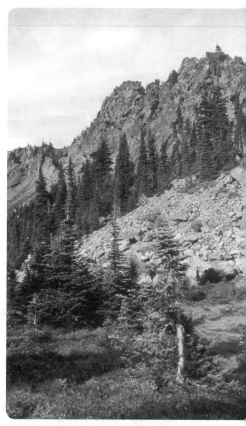

Lemei Rock, Indian Heaven Wilderness

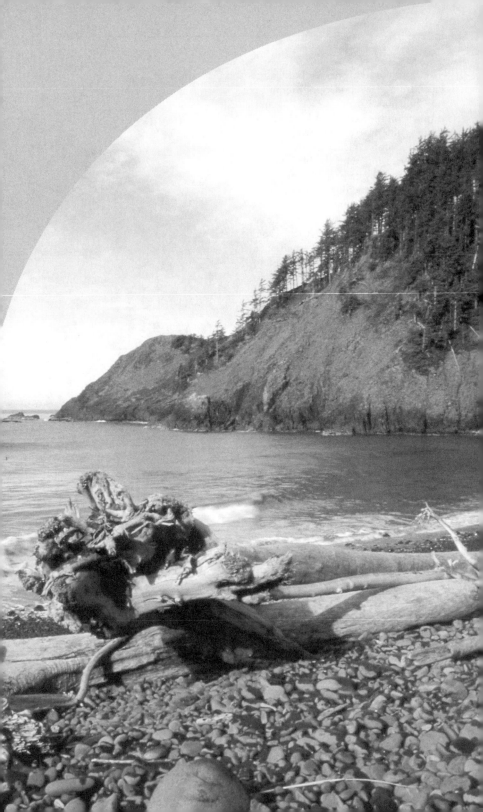

Oregon Coast and Coast Range

The dramatic north coast of Oregon is a land of rugged headlands, off-shore rocks, abundant wildlife, sandy beaches, and generally excellent scenery. Given all that, it is not surprising that the coast attracts lots of tourists. But while the roadside parks are thronged during the summer, those same locations receive very few people in the off-season, and hikers can always escape the worst of the crowds by hitting the trails. Most coastal trails are either too short or have no camping options for backpackers, but there are at least two excellent places where the overnight hiker can combine coastal scenery with a night under the stars, listening to the sound of crashing waves. In the Coast Range, backpacking options are also fairly limited, with only a few hiking destinations that have reasonable camping available. With a little perseverance, however, it is possible to find trails to campsites along salmon streams or at the handful of small lakes hidden amid the dense forests and rugged ridges of these mountains. The lower elevations of the coast and Coast Range provide excellent options for backpackers looking for places to visit in the off-season, when the Cascades Mountains are still covered in a thick blanket of white.

Indian Point from Indian Beach, Ecola State Park (Trip 25)

25 Tillamook Head

RATINGS	Scenery **6** Difficulty **4 to 5** Solitude **4**
ROUND-TRIP DISTANCE	3 miles (from the south); 8.8 miles (from the north)
ELEVATION GAIN	820 feet (from the south); 1200 feet (from the north)
OPTIONAL MAP	*USGS: Tillamook Head*
USUALLY OPEN	All year (but very muddy in winter)
BEST TIMES	March to June
AGENCY	Ecola State Park
PERMIT	None required to camp, but you must purchase a state park day-use pass for each day of your trip (including the day you hike out). Passes cost $3 per day as of 2008. Place the passes on your dashboard and write "Hiker Camp" on them so park rangers know that your vehicle is permitted to park at the trailhead overnight.

Highlights

Tillamook Head is a towering headland that rises more than 1000 feet above the pounding surf of the Pacific Ocean between Cannon Beach and Seaside. This imposing landmark is protected in Ecola State Park, truly one of Oregon's "crown jewel" parks. Along a route taken by Captain William Clark, Sacagawea, and other members of the Lewis and Clark Expedition, the park is crossed by an enjoyable and historic section of the Oregon Coast Trail that passes through lush coastal rain forests and visits several fine viewpoints. Unlike most other trails along the Oregon Coast, this one also includes a designated backpacker's campsite, allowing hikers to extend their stay and enjoy the scenery a little longer. The park enforces a three-night maximum for staying at the Hiker's Camp.

WARNING

Signs at the trailhead correctly warn of steep trailside cliffs along this route. Over the years these cliffs have claimed the lives of more than a few unwary hikers and numerous dogs whose owners failed to have the animals on leash. Please be careful to avoid adding to those sobering statistics.

Getting There

Take U.S. Highway 26 about 70 miles northwest from Portland to its junction with U.S. Highway 101.

To reach the north trailhead, go north on Highway 101 for 3.1 miles, and then turn left at a light at the south end of Seaside onto Avenue U. Proceed 0.2 mile, and then turn left (south) on Edgewood Street, which becomes Sunset Boulevard, and continue 1.4 miles to the road-end trailhead across from an apartment complex.

For the south trailhead, go south from the Highway 26/101 junction and drive 2.9 miles to the turnoff for Cannon Beach. Turn right and wind downhill for 0.5 mile to a junction with the signed road into Ecola State Park. Turn right and go 1.7 miles to the pay station and, immediately thereafter, the turnoff for the Ecola Point Picnic Area.

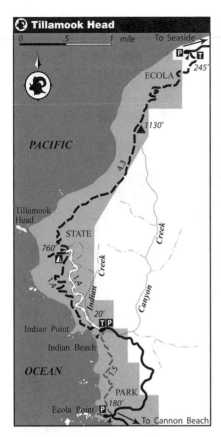

It is possible to start the hike at Ecola Point, but for a shorter route, go right at the junction and drive 1.6 miles to the road-end picnic area and trailhead at Indian Beach. Park officials ask that overnight hikers park at the upper end of the lot, so day users can be near the beach.

Hiking It

Northern Trail: From the north trailhead the signed Oregon Coast Trail sets off through a typically dense coastal rain forest dominated by massive old Douglas firs, western hemlocks, and Sitka spruces. The mossy trunks of

some of these giants rise hundreds of feet into the sky. Beneath this shady canopy the forest floor is covered with salmonberry, sword fern, salal, and hundreds of unusually large deer ferns. The trail goes steadily uphill as it ascends more than a dozen irregularly spaced switchbacks, which help to keep the grade from becoming too steep. Cool ocean breezes make the hike more comfortable and keep you from becoming overheated.

The trail levels off when it rounds the woodsy top of Tillamook Head near 1.7 miles. Several wooden boardwalks here span areas that are prone to becoming muddy. Shortly after you start to go downhill, you come to the hike's first good viewpoint, a high overlook where you can look west over the endless expanse of the Pacific Ocean and south along the precipitous cliffs to a string of offshore rocks. Atop one of the larger rocks, about 1.2 miles out to sea, sits the old Tillamook Rock Lighthouse, which is no longer in service.

The trail now goes up and down (mostly down) through dense woods punctuated by a series of dramatic cliff-edge viewpoints several hundred feet above the crashing waves of the misnamed Pacific Ocean. If you can pry your eyes away from the views, this is a good area to look for bald eagles, which are frequently seen soaring above the headland or perched on trees near the trail.

At 3.8 miles you pass an overlook signed CLARK'S POINT OF VIEW, which Captain William Clark of the Lewis and Clark Expedition considered one of the best he had ever seen. (Perhaps a bit of hyperbole there, Bill, but it is certainly nice.) From here you descend a series of short switchbacks and come to a four-way junction with an old gravel

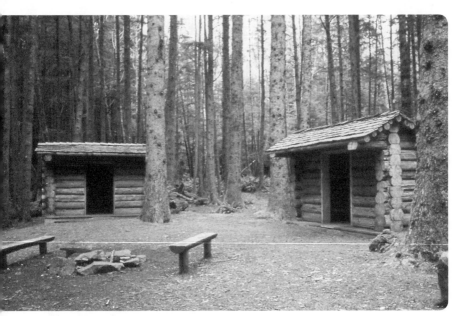

Hiker's Camp along Oregon Coast Trail, Ecola State Park

service road. Turn right and walk 50 yards to the designated Hiker's Camp, complete with three sturdy log shelters with wooden sleeping platforms, a covered picnic table, a fire grate, and an outhouse. The shelters are comfortable and provide protection from the rain, but they are available only on a first-come, first-served basis. Another option is to set up your tent in one of the flat areas a little to the west of the shelters. Beware of mice around the camp and guard your food accordingly. Finding water near the camp is difficult. There is a tiny seasonal creek a bit to the east, but it cannot be relied upon, especially in summer. The best plan is to pack in any water you will need.

The trail continues west for another 0.15 mile, leading downhill past the remains of an abandoned military fortification to yet another stunning viewpoint of Tillamook Rock Lighthouse.

Southern Trail: If you are approaching along the shorter trail from the south, take the Clatsop Loop Trail that begins next to the restroom building at Indian Beach and walk north along an abandoned gravel road. Twisted Sitka spruce trees beside the trail frame photogenic views of Indian Beach to the west. After just 80 yards you come to a junction and the start of a loop.

Go straight, staying on the old gravel road, cross tiny Indian Creek, and soon enter a dark "forest primeval" of tall Sitka spruces and western hemlocks. Salmonberry bushes, sword ferns, oxalis, and other shrubs and wildflowers carpet the forest floor. The old road/trail goes steadily uphill at a moderate grade and passes numerous numbered markers that an interpretive brochure (available at the trailhead) translates into interesting information about this area's natural and human history.

At 1.4 miles the trail abruptly stops climbing, makes a sharp left turn, and proceeds west 150 yards to a signed four-way junction. The Oregon Coast Trail (the northern approach described above) goes right, the return route of the Clatsop Loop goes left, and straight ahead is Hiker's Camp.

For variety on the return, take the western leg of the Clatsop Loop Trail, which goes south from the four-way junction just east of Hiker's Camp. This circuitous footpath goes up and down through dense forest for 0.2 mile and then begins a steady downhill. A series of six switchbacks descend through increasingly open forests and past a small brushy meadow to a pair of excellent viewpoints of rugged Tillamook Head to the north and Tillamook Rock Lighthouse to the west. After a bit more downhill you reach another fine viewpoint, this one complete with a comfortable bench. From here you can look south to Indian Beach, distant Ecola Point, and numerous off-shore rocks, including one prominent arch. The trail finishes its journey by going 0.1 mile down to a bridge over Indian Creek and the close of the loop at the junction with the old road. Turn right to return to the trailhead.

26 Cape Falcon to Short Sand Beach

RATINGS	Scenery **7** Difficulty **5** Solitude **4**
ROUND-TRIP DISTANCE	11.8 miles (including 0.4-mile side trip to Cape Falcon); 6.3 miles (point-to-point)
ELEVATION GAIN	1800 feet; 750 feet (point-to-point)
OPTIONAL MAP	*USGS: Arch Cape*
USUALLY OPEN	All year
BEST TIMES	Any
AGENCY	Oswald West State Park
PERMIT	Required to camp. Permits are available at the campground for $10 per site (as of 2008).

Highlights

Dramatically scenic Oswald West State Park honors one of the giants of the conservation movement in Oregon, a former governor who in the early 20th century had the foresight to set aside all of the state's beaches for public access. The park's most popular attraction is Short Sand Beach, a small but lovely strip of sand hidden away in Smuggler Cove and bordered by the towering cliffs of Cape Falcon. The park operates a unique walk-in campground in the forests above the beach that is designed so that travelers on busy Highway 101 can carry in their overnight gear and have a wilder experience than is usually possible at more developed car campgrounds. Backpackers, who hike in on the outstandingly scenic Oregon Coast Trail, are welcome to spend the night here as well, benefiting from such comforts of home as flush toilets and piped water, but still enjoying a definite wilderness feeling. Since the park is quite popular, it is better to time your visit for midweek or the off-season.

Getting There

Take U.S. Highway 26 about 70 miles northwest from Portland to its junction with U.S. Highway 101. Go south on Highway 101 and drive 12.3 miles to a junction with paved Falcon Cove Road near Milepost 37.2. Turn right (west) and park after 50 yards at the unsigned crossing of the Oregon Coast Trail. There is room here for only about three vehicles. If it is full, you can park at a much larger pull-out along Highway 101 about 0.4 mile north of its junction with Falcon Cove Road, where the Oregon Coast Trail crosses that busy highway.

If you are making this a point-to-point hike, drive the second car 2.1 miles south on Highway 101 and park in the overnight camper's parking lot for Oswald West State Park.

Hiking It

The trail starts in a typical Coast Range forest dominated by second-growth western hemlocks towering over a lush understory of salmonberry, sword fern, salal, and a green mat of mosses. For the first 0.5 mile the path meanders along, going up and down, crossing small ravines on wooden bridges, and passing boggy areas crowded with skunk cabbage. The trail is often muddy in winter, but never steep or overly difficult. Although the forest looks very wild, you are never far from Highway 101, and will often hear traffic zipping by on that busy thoroughfare. As the trail gradually pulls away from the highway, however, the sounds of birds singing, wind in the trees, and wood-

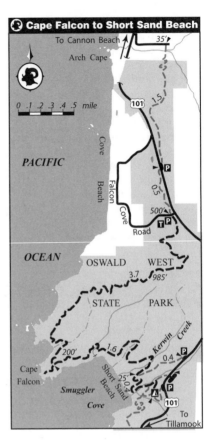

peckers drilling provide a closer match to the wild look of the surroundings.

At 0.6 mile the trail begins an intermittent ascent that leads in two switchbacks to a 985-foot high point on a heavily forested knoll. For the next 0.5 mile the trail goes gradually up and down through terrain that is not only viewless but downright claustrophobic, as you spend most of the time in a living tunnel formed by overhanging tree limbs, salal and rhododendron branches, and salmonberry runners. As you continue going mostly west and enter an old-growth Sitka spruce forest, there are occasional breaks in the greenery that provide views to the southwest of the Pacific Ocean's endless blue expanse.

The trail then descends, winding steadily downhill in more open forest to a fine viewpoint of the rugged coastline to the north. Over the next 0.6 mile the downhill continues and takes you past several unmarked side trails that quickly lead to dramatic viewpoints atop crumbling cliffs that are hundreds of feet above the surf. Do not go too far out on these points, however, because they are often eroded underneath and quite unstable. At a switchback at 3.3 miles an obvious 20-yard side trail goes straight to a particularly stunning

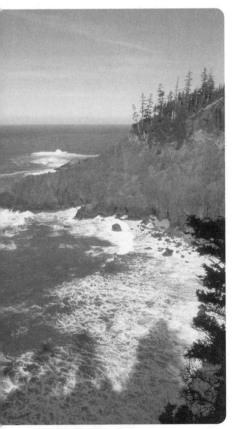

Cliffs north of Cape Falcon

viewpoint overlooking a wave-pounded cove on the north side of Cape Falcon. In the spring, you can use binoculars to scan the ocean here for migrating gray whales or look down to the water to see dozens of pigeon guillemots. These sleek, jet-black diving birds have large white wing patches and breed by the thousands along the Oregon coast.

The trail goes inland from this viewpoint to a hop-over crossing of the small creek that empties into the cove. The scenery then becomes increasingly dramatic as you go past fine viewpoints on your way out to the prominent headland of Cape Falcon. At 3.7 miles is an unsigned but obvious junction in an area of dense, head-high salal bushes. Unless the weather is *really* bad (and if it is, what are you doing here?), turn right and follow a dead-end, 0.2-mile side trail up to some outstanding viewpoints atop Cape Falcon. To the south is pyramid-shaped Neahkahnie Mountain, while to the north is a very photogenic rocky coastline. Don't be surprised if you see a bald eagle perched on a rock or tree limb overlooking the ocean. You may also spot whales, seals, sea lions, or even dolphins swimming in the water.

To reach Short Sand Beach, take the heavily traveled trail that goes slightly left at the Cape Falcon junction and head inland through relatively open forests that provide several fine viewpoints looking south to Neahkahnie Mountain. After 0.5 mile you take a bridge over a small creek a little above an unseen waterfall that cascades down onto Short Sand Beach. Just beyond this crossing, you may notice a pair of unmaintained side trails that drop to the right. Although these use paths lead to the beach below, they are wickedly steep and extremely dangerous, especially when wet, so they are best avoided. The well-engineered main trail wanders up and down through forest and over muddy skunk-cabbage bogs to the crossing of an unnamed seasonal creek, and then a hop-over crossing of slightly larger Kerwin Creek before reaching a signed junction at 5.3 miles.

The trail to the left is a spur to Highway 101. Go straight, almost immediately pass a viewpoint of Short Sand Beach, and then descend a switchback to the developed picnic area just above the sand. The beach is very beautiful, with fine views of rugged Cape Falcon to the north. If conditions are right you may also have the opportunity to watch a hardy group of surfers who often come to Short Sand Beach to enjoy their sport.

The picnic area boasts several tables, metal fire grills, a restroom building, and piped water, but camping is not allowed here or on the beach.

To reach the designated camping area, take the wide, gravel-covered trail that goes inland, crosses Short Sand Creek on a bridge, and after 0.1 mile reaches a junction with the southbound Oregon Coast Trail. Go straight, walk another 0.1 mile, and then turn right and continue 150 yards to the signed camping area. Here you will find many amenities unfamiliar to most backpackers, including numbered sites, piped water, flush toilets, and garbage collection, all catering to the walk-in campers from nearby Highway 101. There is also a self-registration pay station where you are required to obtain a permit and pay your $10 per site fee. The park enforces a 6-person-per-site limit and requires that all dogs be on leash. To reach the overnight camper's parking lot, follow the trail that departs from the south side of the camping area and climbs 0.2 mile to the road.

27 Soapstone Lake

RATINGS	Scenery **5** Difficulty **1** Solitude **9**
ROUND-TRIP DISTANCE	2.4 miles (including loop around lake)
ELEVATION GAIN	250 feet
OPTIONAL MAP	*USGS: Soapstone Lake* (trail not shown)
USUALLY OPEN	All year (except during winter storms)
BEST TIMES	April to November
AGENCY	Clatsop State Forest
PERMIT	None

Highlights

The recently completed trail to Soapstone Lake is a pleasant and easy backpacking outing that makes an excellent choice for families with children. The trail to the lake is short but surprisingly diverse, including areas of dense forest, some relatively open second-growth woodlands, a small meadow, and a lovely creek, all leading to a pretty lake at trail's end. Wildlife is common and the lake is surprisingly scenic, so there is plenty to appreciate regardless of your age or hiking abilities. Be aware that, since the Clatsop State Forest manages this land as a "working forest," hikers should expect periodic trail closures due to timber harvest activity. Call ahead for the latest conditions.

Getting There

Go west on U.S. Highway 26 from Portland to the junction with State Highway 53 near Milepost 9.5. Turn left (south), drive 4.8 miles, and then turn left on a gravel road signed SOAP- STONE TRAILHEAD. Proceed 0.4 mile on the narrow road to the signed trailhead and parking area.

Hiking It

The wide, smooth, and gently graded trail travels through a second-growth forest dominated by western hemlocks towering above a thick mat of oxalis, various ferns, and thimbleberry bushes. Several huge stumps with old logging springboard holes attest that the forest here was once composed of much larger specimens. Much of this lower trail is scheduled for harvest again in 2008, so expect to encounter logging scars for the next several years. The trail crosses two often-dry creeks on wooden bridges, and then at 0.3 mile gradually loses a little elevation before crossing a small grassy meadow where a homestead was once located. In late summer this meadow delights the visitor with ripe blackberries and blooming goldenrods. During the winter and early spring you may see elk here, especially in the early morning.

At the far end of the meadow is a crossing of clear Soapstone Creek. This crossing currently requires a ford but there are plans to install a log bridge in the future. After the crossing, you climb a rather steep set of wooden

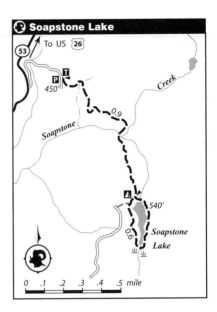

stairs and then wander uphill through a lovely forest of impressive old Douglas firs before coming to a T junction near the north end of Soapstone Lake. To reach the lake's best campsite, turn right at the junction and walk 50 yards uphill to a spacious and comfortable site on the left.

The lake is fun to explore, and a trail going all the way around its shore makes this easy. A clockwise tour takes you over a bridge spanning the outlet creek and past several inviting picnic spots to a fine little rocky beach near a beaver lodge along the east shore. This is a good spot to fish for cutthroat trout or for kids to observe the lake's abundant population of roughskin newts. From here the loop trail continues to a boardwalk over a skunk-cabbage bog at the lake's south end, and then goes up and down along the west shore to a junction with a trail to a nearby logging road. Turn right and walk a few yards downhill to the campsite and the trail back to your car.

28 North Fork Salmonberry River

RATINGS	Scenery **5** Difficulty **2** Solitude **9**
ROUND-TRIP DISTANCE	4.2 miles (or more, depending on how far you can drive on the rough access road)
ELEVATION GAIN	840 feet
OPTIONAL MAP	*Tillamook State Forest*
USUALLY OPEN	All year
BEST TIMES	Late March to mid-May
AGENCY	Tillamook State Forest
PERMIT	None

Highlights

Although the access road is rough and challenging, this hike into a remote canyon in the rain forests of Oregon's Coast Range is a real winner. The clear North Fork Salmonberry River is not only beautiful to look at but it is an important spawning stream for runs of salmon and steelhead. In fact, at a small falls along the trail from mid-March to mid-May, you can often observe these magnificent fish leaping over the falls on their way upstream. Added to the usual treats of a lovely, moss-draped forest and a pretty stream to camp beside, this wildlife show makes spring the best time to visit this little-known retreat.

Getting There

Drive U.S. Highway 26 west from Portland to an obscure junction just 0.4 mile west of Milepost 32. Turn left (south) on signed gravel Salmonberry Road and proceed 1.3 miles to a four-way junction. Go straight, still on Salmonberry Road, and stay on the main road for 2.8 miles through several minor intersections to a junction. Turn

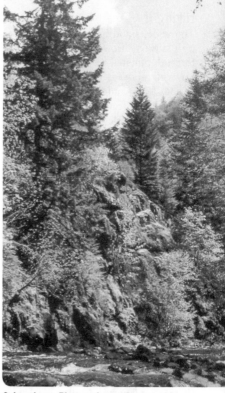

Salmonberry River at the confluence with North Folk

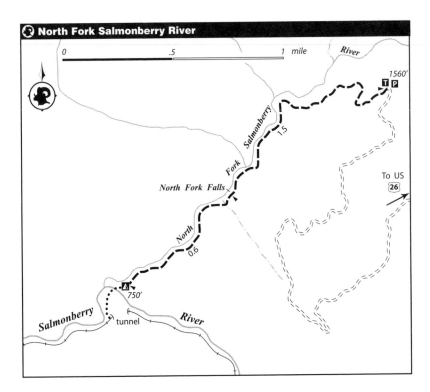

North Fork Salmonberry River

left, then veer right just 20 yards later onto a road that soon become a rough gravel route with a high center, requiring a vehicle with good ground clearance to negotiate. When conditions are wet, this road can be extremely difficult for passenger cars without four-wheel drive. Continue 4.7 miles to another four-way junction, go straight, and remain on this narrow, rough, and often steeply downhill road for 4.5 miles to a berm that blocks further motorized travel.

Hiking It

On the other side of the berm the route follows the closed jeep road, now long abandoned and overgrown with grasses, ferns, and alders. The surrounding forest is the usual lush Coast Range

mix of western hemlocks, red alders, bigleaf maples, and Douglas firs. Just to the right (west) of your route flow the joyfully cascading waters of the stunningly beautiful North Fork Salmonberry River. The walk is easy and pleasant, with the road lined by tall, white-barked red alder trees and spreading bigleaf maples, with lots of perky forest wildflowers below.

At 1.5 miles you encounter North Fork Falls, where the stream drops over a pair of low basalt ledges into a rocky chasm. Although the falls is less than 10 feet high, that is just the right height to force migrating fish to make spectacular leaps to reach the top. The show is impressive to watch, even though you may have to wait several minutes between fishy high-jump attempts. While waiting for these athletic leaps, you can amuse yourself by watching the little gray dippers that nest along this stream.

About 0.6 mile below North Fork Falls, just above the confluence of the North Fork and the main stem Salmonberry River, the old road ends at a grassy flat. This is a good place to set up camp and enjoy the lush canyon and river scenery. For a longer outing, it is possible to extend this adventure by fording the Salmonberry River (usually only knee deep after the rainy season ends) and then scrambling up to the tracks of the Tillamook Railroad on the other side. From here you can walk for miles either upstream or down, visiting abandoned railroad towns, checking out tall railroad trestles, and walking through tunnels. Just be careful of trains, especially in the dark and narrow tunnels where there is no room to get off the tracks to avoid oncoming locomotives.

Columbia River Gorge

Cutting a nearly sea-level canyon through one of North America's greatest mountain ranges, the mighty Columbia River has created a scenic treasure right at Portland's doorstep. The Columbia River Gorge (or simply "The Gorge," as locals refer to it) is a land of countless waterfalls, towering cliffs, howling winds, and dramatic scenery. The Gorge's east-west orientation provides for strikingly different vegetation zones, as in just 50 miles you move from lush rain forests in the west to a treeless desert of sagebrush and dry grasses in the east. Hiking in this vertical landscape is often challenging, but highly rewarding. Possible overnight destinations include not only the familiar stream canyons and waterfalls of places like Eagle Creek but also remote lakes in the forested mountains both north and south of the river, as well as high ridges with excellent views of the rugged canyonlands below. Amazingly, some of the best trails are less than an hour's drive from downtown Portland. It is easy to see why the Gorge has been a popular local outdoor destination for over 100 years.

29 Silver Star Mountain

RATINGS	Scenery **8** Difficulty **4 to 7** Solitude **6**
ROUND-TRIP DISTANCE	5.6 miles for north loop; 13.5 miles for Bluff Mountain Trail
ELEVATION GAIN	1700 feet for north loop; 2600 feet for Bluff Mountain Trail
OPTIONAL MAPS	*Green Trails: Bridal Veil, Lookout Mountain*
USUALLY OPEN	Mid-May to mid-November
BEST TIMES	Mid-June to Mid-July
AGENCY	Mount St. Helens National Volcanic Monument
PERMIT	None

Highlights

As seen from Portland, Silver Star Mountain is that long, brownish ridge to the northeast that frustratingly blocks the view of Mt. Adams. But from atop this ridge there is nothing to obstruct the views, not only of Mt. Adams, but of pretty much everything else for 50 or more miles in any direction. And it's not just the views that make a visit here worthwhile. In 1902, the massive Yacolt Burn swept over this peak, killing nearly all the trees. The forests have yet to return, so despite its relatively low elevation, the peak has an open, almost alpine appearance, with plenty of sunshine to nourish thousands of acres of wildflowers in June and July. Surprisingly few hikers visit this area, and those that do almost always make it a dayhike. But a campsite near a little-known spring just southwest of the summit allows backpackers to spend the night, watch a terrific sunset, and even see the lights of Portland twinkling far below. Several routes lead to the summit, and every one of them is outstanding. The two best are a relatively short but very attractive loop from the north and a longer and even more scenic trail from the east.

Getting There

From the intersection of State Highways 502 and 503 in downtown Battleground, Washington, drive 5.7 miles north on Highway 503 to a junction. Turn right on N.E. Rock Creek Road, which soon becomes Lucia Falls Road, and proceed 8.6 miles to a junction. Turn right on Sunset Falls Road and drive 7.4 miles to a junction at the entrance to Sunset Campground. Turn right on gravel Forest Road 41 and almost immediately cross a bridge to an unsigned junction where you go left. Proceed 3.5 miles on this pothole-filled road to an unsigned junction with Road 4109.

If you are taking the shorter northern loop trail, turn sharply right (downhill) on Road 4109 and stay on this sometimes rough road for 1.5 miles to a multiway junction. Turn left and go 2.7 steep, bumpy, uphill miles to the road-end turnaround and trailhead.

If you plan to take the Bluff Mountain Trail from the east, continue straight on Road 41 from its junction with Road 4109 and proceed 5.5 miles to the trailhead at a prominent open saddle. Parking is on the right.

Hiking It

Northern Loop Option: The signed Silver Star Trail begins by switchbacking four times up a slope covered with brushy vine maple to a junction with a closed jeep road. Bear right (uphill) and walk 150 yards along the road to a large gravel turnaround.

The scenery here, and for some time to come, is outstanding. The entire area is surrounded by huge sloping meadows that are carpeted with wildflowers in late June and early July. There are dozens of varieties, but the most common kinds are beargrass, lupine, wild carrot, paintbrush, iris, yarrow, valerian, tiger lily, and golden pea. Scattered about the open slopes are perky little noble and Pacific silver fir trees.

In addition to the flowers and trees, there are terrific views. Most impressive are Mt. St. Helens and Mt. Rainier, peeking over forested ridges to the north, and Mt. Adams to the east. Southward, Mt. Hood makes an almost perfectly framed appearance in a low point in the ridge east of Silver Star Mountain.

If you are making the recommended loop, you will return on the old jeep road that goes to the right. For now, bear left at a sign identifying Ed's Trail, and follow this rough and narrow but extremely scenic route as it steeply ascends near the edge of a drop-off. The huge meadows here boast even more flowers than those you passed below. Added to the previous mix are columbine, wallflower, penstemon, fireweed, lomatium, and bistort, all looking for

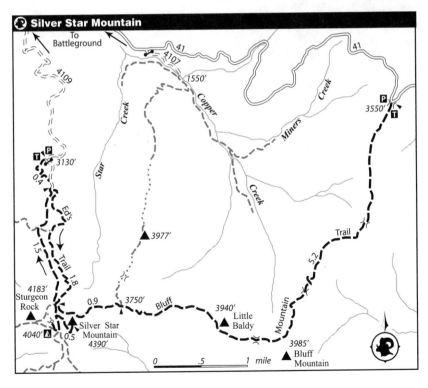

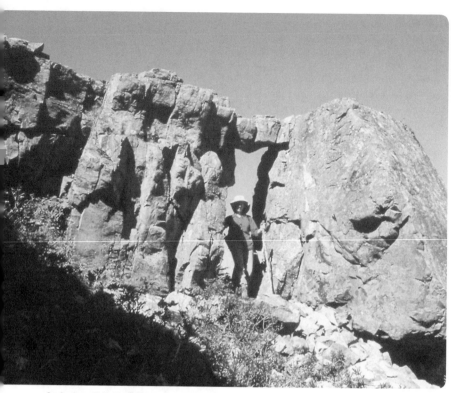

Arch along Ed's Trail, Silver Star Mountain

their place among the other blossoms. After the trail rounds a small ridge, the scenery improves yet again as the rocky spine of Silver Star Mountain's summit ridge becomes visible directly ahead.

Still crossing mostly open slopes, you climb gradually to the ridge crest, where you meet an ancient two-rut road. Turn left, and in just 100 feet you come to a possibly unsigned junction with a trail going down to the right. Continue straight and keep climbing as the trail skirts to the left of several jagged rock outcroppings on the spine of the ridge. Along one of these detours, you go through a natural, keyhole-shaped rock arch.

Shortly after the arch, the trail goes very steeply up some improvised rock steps, where you may have to use your hands to help pull yourself up. Dogs will have a very difficult time negotiating this section. At the top of this short but difficult climb, you go through a notch in the cliff and then descend through a very scenic, flower-filled meadow. Once the trail leaves the meadow, it enters a forest of Pacific silver fir and soon comes to a major ridgetop junction.

The jeep road you have been paralleling meets your route here, as does the Bluff Mountain Trail (the alternate approach trail from the east), which angles in from the left. There is also an unsigned trail directly across the road, which goes southwest toward Sturgeon Rock.

Turn left (south) on the jeep route and climb for 200 yards to a road junction. To reach the summit, bear left and ascend a rock-strewn old road for about 0.2 mile to the high saddle between the twin summits of Silver Star Mountain. The north summit is slightly higher and has better views. On very clear days you can see not only the nearby volcanic peaks already mentioned but also south to Mt. Jefferson and the Three Sisters in Oregon, and northwest to Washington's Olympic Mountains.

To reach the campsite, return to the junction 0.2 mile below the summit and go south (downhill) along a jeep track for 0.2 mile to a junction. Turn right, walk 50 yards, then turn right again onto an unsigned but obvious trail. This path goes 80 yards to a small but reliable piped spring with a fine nearby campsite.

To make a loop on the way back, return to the ridgetop junction a little north of the summit of Silver Star Mountain, where the Bluff Mountain Trail and Ed's Trail meet the jeep road. Instead of walking back on Ed's Trail, take the jeep road as it gently descends for 1.9 miles through view-packed meadows and past rock formations back to the trailhead.

Eastern Option: The Bluff Mountain Trail starts as an old jeep road, now closed to motor vehicles, that undulates along a scenic, mostly open ridgetop.

The route provides extensive views and is carpeted with a delightful mix of small Pacific silver fir trees, huckleberry and serviceberry bushes, beargrass, and a wide array of wildflowers.

After 2 up-and-down miles, you descend to a small saddle where the road ends and the trail veers to the right. From here the path loses more elevation in one long switchback to another, more prominent saddle, and then cuts across the north side of Bluff Mountain, where in early summer you may encounter lingering snow patches and small runoff creeks. After completing the traverse, the trail climbs to and crosses another saddle, this one in dense timber, and then traverses the open, view-packed talus slopes on the south and west sides of pyramid-shaped Little Baldy. Here you'll have great views of the impressive crags of Silver Star Mountain to the west. Still traveling toward that goal, the well-graded trail uses two short switchbacks to work its way gradually up an open ridge with lots of beargrass.

Go straight at the signed junction with the rarely-used Starway Trail, and then climb through the forest on the north side of Silver Star Mountain, where snowdrifts usually remain into late June. The trail ends at a multiway intersection, where you encounter a closed jeep road and Ed's Trail. Turn left and follow the directions to the summit and the campsite described above.

30 | Soda Peaks Lake

RATINGS	Scenery **6** Difficulty **4** Solitude **7**
ROUND-TRIP DISTANCE	4.6 miles
ELEVATION GAIN	1300 feet
OPTIONAL MAP	*Green Trails: Lookout Mountain*
USUALLY OPEN	June to November
BEST TIMES	Mid-June to early October
AGENCY	Mount Adams Ranger District (Gifford Pinchot National Forest)
PERMIT	Free at the trailhead.

Highlights

Although perhaps not as spectacularly scenic as some of the other lakes described in these pages, Soda Peaks Lake is still very attractive, with its clear, greenish waters backed by an encircling ridge of forests and talus slopes. Trout jump almost continuously, enticing the angler, while the waters are warm enough for swimming by early to mid-July. All in all, this tranquil spot makes a great place for a quiet night in the wilderness.

Getting There

Drive Interstate 84 east to Cascade Locks, take Exit 44, and almost immediately veer right to loop around and cross the Columbia River on the Bridge of the Gods (a $1 toll applies, as of 2008). Turn right on State Highway 14, go 6.1 miles, and then turn left (north) on the signed road to Carson. After 0.9 mile you go straight at a junction in the middle of Carson, and then proceed 7.9 miles to another junction. Turn left, following signs to Wind Riv-

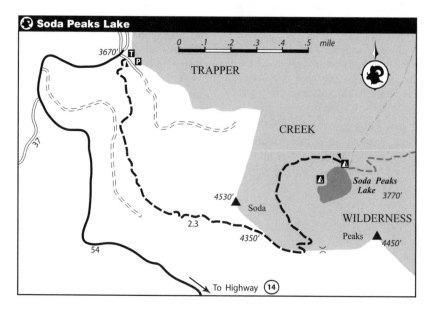

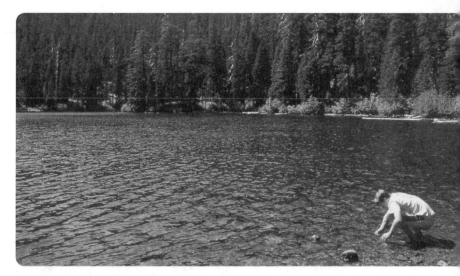

Exploring Soda Peaks Lake, Trapper Creek Wilderness

er Visitors Center, and go 0.3 mile to a four-way junction. Turn right on Szydlo (yes, that's spelled correctly) Road, which later narrows to one-lane pavement when it becomes Forest Road 54. Go 13.3 miles, staying on Road 54 at all intersections, to a four-way junction at the end of pavement. Turn right and almost immediately park near a large trailhead signboard.

Hiking It

The trail begins in a small, regrowing clear-cut, but soon enters an attractive uncut forest of stately hemlocks and firs. Huckleberry bushes, avalanche lilies, and beargrass are among the most common of the abundant plants crowding the forest floor. In the first 0.3 mile the up-and-down trail skirts a couple of old clear-cuts, the second of which opens up a terrific view of Mt. Adams to the northeast. After this you reenter woods and begin a steady, moderately steep climb. The route closely follows an east-west oriented ridgeline nearly

to the top of the western summit of the two Soda Peaks, and then cuts across the forested south side of that peak to arrive at an open ridgetop viewpoint. From here you can look north to such snowy landmarks as Mt. Rainier and the Goat Rocks, as well as down to the shimmering waters of Soda Peaks Lake.

To reach the lake, the trail descends nearly to the saddle between the two Soda Peaks, and then makes a sharp left turn to begin its descent of the north side of the ridge. You switchback twice down the heavily forested hillside as the trail winds gradually down to a very roomy campsite near the outlet on the north shore of Soda Peaks Lake. Views to the ridge rising above the south shore are very attractive and make a nice backdrop for an evening meal. The lake is fun for youngsters to explore, since the water is reasonably warm and has lots of trout, crayfish, and newts to keep kids interested.

31 Dublin Lake and Tanner Butte

RATINGS	Scenery **7** Difficulty **7 to 9** Solitude **7**
ROUND-TRIP DISTANCE	13.8 miles to Dublin Lake; 22.4 miles to Tanner Lake
ELEVATION GAIN	4200 feet to Dublin Lake; 4700 feet to Tanner Lake
OPTIONAL MAP	*Green Trails: Bonneville Dam*
USUALLY OPEN	Late May to October
BEST TIMES	June
AGENCY	Columbia River Gorge National Scenic Area
PERMIT	None. Northwest Forest Pass required.

Highlights

The bulky mass of Tanner Butte, with its gouged-out eastern face, is a well-known landmark in the central Columbia River Gorge. Given its prominence, it is not surprising that the summit features stupendous views of distant, snow-covered peaks, as well as the surrounding deep canyons, rugged ridges, and dense forests. But the hike to Tanner Butte offers much more than a nice view at the end. The forests here are varied, beautiful, and interesting. The open ridge north of Tanner Butte has outstanding wildflower displays in June. The trail is surprisingly uncrowded. And near the mountain are fine camps, either beside a small spring or, for those up for a bit of off-trail scrambling, at a very scenic little lake directly beneath Tanner Butte's cliffs and talus slopes. For hikers who prefer an easier destination, forest-rimmed Dublin Lake is a good goal.

Getting There

Leave Interstate 84 at Exit 40, turn right (south) at the bottom of the exit ramp, and immediately come to a T junction. Bear right and go about 100 yards to the parking lot for Wahclella Falls Trail.

Hiking It

Walk back to the T junction in the road and pick up the eastbound Gorge Trail as it climbs in switchbacks and traverses a forested hillside. After about 0.8 mile, the trail follows a power line access road for 0.2 mile to a junction with the closed Tanner Creek Road, where you turn right. Walk this road uphill as it rounds a ridge and enters the canyon of Tanner Creek. At 2.2 miles the signed Tanner Butte Trail leaves from the left side of the road, just before you cross a small creek in a side canyon.

The trail goes up a lush little canyon with several small waterfalls, crossing two branches of the creek before climbing through forest and twice going under a power line. You cross the rough power line access road at a diagonal, and then go up a series of 11 switchbacks on a heavily forested hillside. From here the trail makes a long traverse to a dry campsite and ridge crest junction where the unofficial Wauna Point Trail goes to the left.

Keep right, staying on the main trail, and begin a long, moderately graded ascent of a wide forested ridge. There are no views along the way, but the hiking is never tedious, as the forest

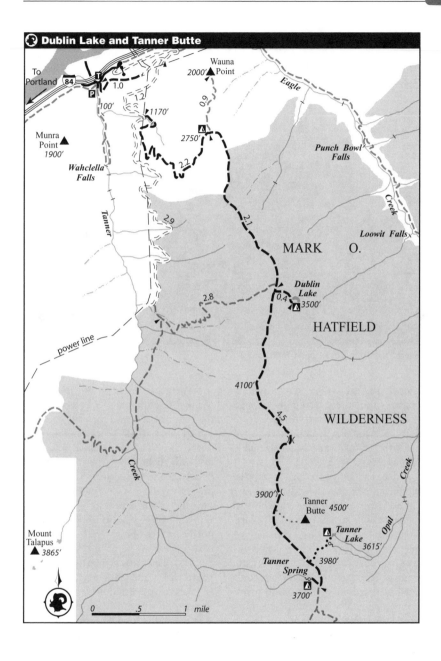

Dublin Lake and Tanner Butte

To Portland 84

Wauna Point 2000'

Eagle

Munra Point 1900'

Punch Bowl Falls

Wahclella Falls

2750'

2.2

1170'

1.0

1.2

100'

0.9

2.9

2.1

Tanner

Loowit Falls

MARK   O.

Dublin Lake 3500'

0.4

2.8

HATFIELD

power line

4100'

4.5

WILDERNESS

Creek

3900'

Tanner Butte 4500'

Opal Creek

Tanner Lake 3615'

Mount Talapus 3865'

Tanner Spring 3980'

3700'

0   .5   1 mile

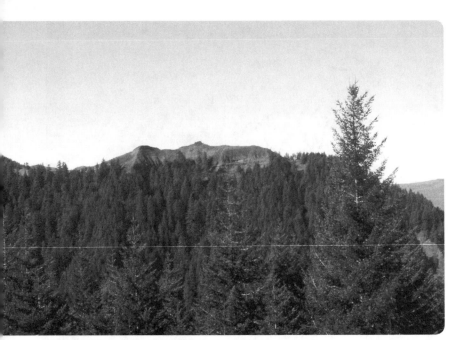

Munra Point from Tanner Butte Trail

is open and attractive. As you gain elevation, the forest gradually changes to a typical mid-elevation type, dominated by Douglas fir and Pacific silver fir, with lots of beargrass and huckleberries on the forest floor.

At 6.5 miles you come to a possibly unsigned junction with the Tanner Cutoff Trail, which goes downhill to the right. Go straight and, 150 yards later, reach the junction with the 0.4-mile spur trail to Dublin Lake. If this lake is your goal, then turn left and begin a steep downhill that leads to the northwest corner of this small, forest-rimmed pool. The best place to camp is above the southwest shore.

Although Dublin Lake is isolated and serene, it is not especially scenic. For better scenery, return to the Tanner Butte Trail and go south as the trail wanders lazily along the wide ridge and

soon drops to meet an old jeep road. Make a careful note of where you meet the road, as the trail turnoff is poorly signed on the way back. Follow this overgrown road for 1 mile, and then descend slightly to where the forest opens up and the scenery abruptly improves. To the east, you can look down into the green depths of Eagle Creek Canyon, while due south is the steep northeast face of massive Tanner Butte. At your feet are acres of colorful wildflowers, especially beargrass, lupine, paintbrush, and larkspur. The road is overgrown with huckleberries and foot-tripping beargrass, but the scenery is so good it is hard to complain.

Still on the old road, continue south through increasingly open and attractive meadows and rocky slopes, and then go over a view-packed knoll to a wide saddle on the north side of Tanner

Butte. If you want to reach the summit, leave the road at the saddle and scramble cross-country up the northwest side of the peak. Try not to get too close to the steep drop-off on your left, because the rocks may be unstable. The first few hundred yards are rather difficult, as you have to fight through some brush, but then the going improves as the country opens up. From the top the views extend to Mounts St. Helens, Adams, and Rainier in Washington, as well as Mt. Hood in Oregon. Hikers familiar with the area can identify countless other lesser landmarks, such as Washington's Silver Star Mountain and Oregon's Larch and Chinidere mountains.

There are two possible campsites in this area, both south of Tanner Butte. To reach them, follow the trail as it curves around the brushy west side of Tanner Butte and comes to a ridge just south of the peak. To reach Tan-

ner Lake, turn left (east) off the trail and scramble down a fairly steep and forested slope into the cirque basin that holds this scenic little lake. The way down is brushy, but not terribly difficult. The view across the lake up to the rugged cliffs of Tanner Butte makes the cross-country travel worthwhile. If you prefer to camp at Tanner Spring, continue on the trail going south, walk about 0.3 mile, and then look for a possibly unsigned trail that goes sharply right. This spur trail goes 0.2 mile to Tanner Spring, where there is a nice campsite. This spur trail is not regularly maintained, so you should expect some deadfall.

You can return the way you came, or, if you are feeling ambitious, you can turn this into an exciting 28-mile loop by descending east along the steep Eagle-Tanner Trail and walking back to civilization along the scenic and popular Eagle Creek Trail (see Trip 32).

32 Eagle Creek

RATINGS	Scenery **9** Difficulty **3 to 6** Solitude **2**
ROUND-TRIP DISTANCE	8 miles to Tenas Camp; 16.8 miles to the last creekside campsite (with many intermediate options)
ELEVATION GAIN	750 feet to Tenas Camp; 1700 feet to the last creekside campsite
OPTIONAL MAP	*Green Trails: Bonneville Dam*
USUALLY OPEN	All year (except during winter storms)
BEST TIMES	April to October
AGENCY	Columbia River Gorge National Scenic Area
PERMIT	Required. Free at the wilderness boundary. Northwest Forest Pass required.

Highlights

The Eagle Creek Trail has been a favorite of local hikers since it was first built in 1915. The trail opened at the same time as the Old Columbia River Scenic Highway, providing a spectacular hiking destination for visitors just discovering the area. Today, it remains one of the most outstanding and popular trails in our region, leading hikers through a

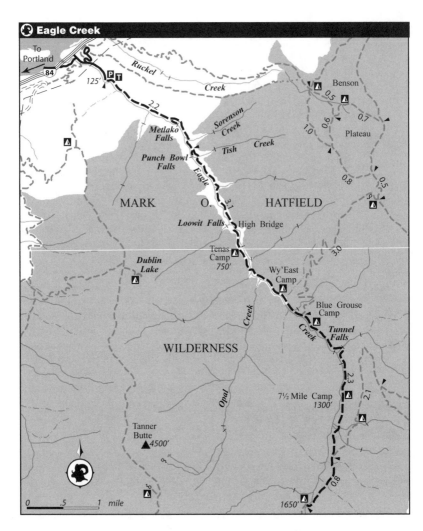

Eagle Creek

verdant canyon, beside waterfalls in every shape and size, and along a creek that is almost unbelievably beautiful. To protect the resource, the U.S. Forest Service requires that you camp only in designated sites, prohibits fires within 200 feet of the trail, and asks that you leave your dog at home. The steep drop-offs found along parts of this trail make it unsuitable for young children.

Getting There

Leave the eastbound lanes of Interstate 84 at Exit 41, turn right (south) at the bottom of the exit road, and drive 0.6 mile to the parking lot at the end of the road. Parking is often full on summer weekends, so try to arrive early. Leave nothing of value in your car, as break-ins have been a problem here for years. As an alternative, you might want to park in the lot behind the fish hatchery at the bottom of the exit ramp and walk 0.6 mile up the road to the trailhead.

Hiking It

The trail begins with a gradual uphill on a wooded hillside above the cascading stream. After a brief stint in the bottomlands, the path crosses some very steep slopes a few hundred feet above the creek that afford you nice views down into the canyon. Along the way it crosses several small, unnamed side creeks, which add variety to the lush forest scenery. Poison oak is part of that lush vegetation, but the wide, heavily used trail makes avoiding the plant easy.

At 1.5 miles a short side trail to the right makes a loop past a fenced overlook, where you can look up a narrow canyon to the impressive drop of Metlako Falls. Not long after this marvelous taste of things to come, you cross small Sorenson Creek on a bridge and come to a junction with a side trail going to the bottom of Punch Bowl Falls. Don't miss the chance to visit this short but spectacular waterfall. For decades calendars have featured this outstanding scene, with a glassy creek winding through a fern-lined grotto where a perfect bowl-shaped falls drops into a pool at the head of the canyon.

Back on the main trail, you traverse heavily wooded slopes to a viewpoint directly above Punch Bowl Falls, giving you a different perspective of this classic cascade. Above this point, the scenery grows even more dramatic, as you are forced to cross vertical basalt cliffs where the trail has been blasted into the side of the rock. Along one of these steep slopes you get a terrific view of wispy Loowit Falls, on a side creek across the canyon. Shortly after this, you cross appropriately named High Bridge, which spans a slot canyon about 90 feet above the clear waters of Eagle Creek.

After the bridge the slopes are less steep, and are covered with dense forests. At Tenas Camp (4 miles), the first legal campsite along the creek, you may want to take a side trip to the creek to visit a lovely two-tiered

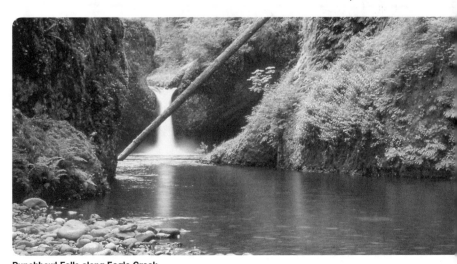

Punchbowl Falls along Eagle Creek

waterfall, which has very nice pools near its base that invite a *cold* dip in the water. Above Tenas Camp, you recross the creek on a bridge, and then work your way upstream to Wy'East Camp (4.9 miles). About 0.3 mile past this camp you come to a junction with the little-used and now overgrown Eagle-Benson Trail.

Keep straight on the main trail and go gradually uphill in partial forest past Blue Grouse Camp (5.4 miles), and then traverse through forest and over talus slopes well above the creek. A steep side trail drops down one of these talus slopes, visiting an impressive waterfall on the creek, but most people skip this attraction and head straight for nearby Tunnel Falls. This colossal, 120-foot-high waterfall drops over a sheer cliff in the shady side canyon of East Fork Eagle Creek. The trail goes behind the falls in a human-made tunnel dynamited out of the cliff about

halfway up. You should expect to get wet, but it's an exhilarating walk.

Just past Tunnel Falls, you round a ridge where the trail once again takes an exposed course blasted out of vertical basalt cliffs right beside another tall falls on the main branch of the creek. Metal cables here give acrophobic hikers something to hang on to and a greater sense of security.

At 6.9 miles you come to misnamed 7½ Mile Camp, which gets far fewer people than the camps lower in the canyon. If you want even more privacy, however, continue another 0.7 mile to a junction with the faint Eagle-Tanner Trail. Go straight and walk gradually uphill through forest another 0.8 mile to a ford of Eagle Creek. There is a fine and little-used campsite here that is a great place to spend the night listening to "river music" and watching cheerful little dippers (small gray birds) as they dive into the cold, rushing water to feed.

33 Herman Creek Trail

RATINGS	Scenery **6** Difficulty **5 to 8** Solitude **7**
ROUND-TRIP DISTANCE	14.6 miles to Cedar Swamp Camp; 19 miles to Mud Lake
ELEVATION GAIN	2850 feet to Cedar Swamp; 3700 feet to Mud Lake
OPTIONAL MAP	*Green Trails: Bonneville Dam*
USUALLY OPEN	Mid-March to November for Cedar Swamp; mid-May to early November for Mud Lake
BEST TIMES	April to June
AGENCY	Columbia River Gorge National Scenic Area
PERMIT	None. Northwest Forest Pass required.

Highlights

Herman Creek is one of the major streams of the Columbia River Gorge, and the trail up its long canyon leads

to a number of interesting and worthwhile destinations. Although the trail generally stays in the forests on the hillside well above cascading Herman

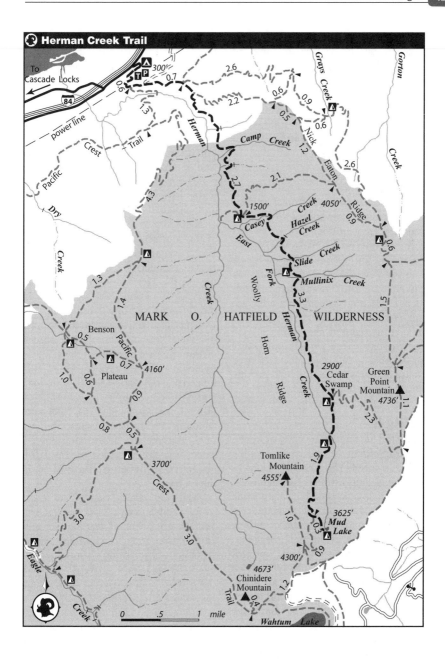

Creek, it passes beneath several tall, wispy waterfalls on side streams, and is much less crowded than the better known Eagle Creek Trail (Trip 32). Backpackers have several options for spending the night, but the best locations are Cedar Swamp Camp and Mud Lake. Both are very attractive and far from any crowds.

Getting There

Take Interstate 84 east from Portland, leaving the freeway at Exit 44 for Cascade Locks. Continue 1.2 miles east through town on the main road (Wa Na Pa Street), and then turn left on Forest Lane at a sign for the airport. Stay on this road for 2 miles, and then turn left at a T junction immediately after going over a freeway overpass. Drive 0.4 mile, turn right at the entrance road for Herman Creek Campground, and go 0.3 mile up this one-lane paved road following signs to the trailhead parking lot.

Hiking It

The trail departs from the west end of the parking lot and winds steadily uphill in several turns and switchbacks through a stately forest of Douglas firs, western hemlocks, and bigleaf and vine maples. At 0.4 mile you pass under a set of power lines, and then continue uphill to a fork at 0.6 mile. Bear left, still on Herman Creek Trail, and proceed gradually up a mostly forested hillside to a switchback in an abandoned dirt road. Bear right and follow this old road as it steadily climbs for 0.4 mile, then levels off before continuing 0.2 mile to a signed junction.

You go straight and travel slightly downhill along a heavily wooded hillside. Swift-flowing Herman Creek can be heard but not seen in the canyon

on your right. At 2.2 miles, you pass beside a tall, lacy waterfall on an unnamed little creek, and shortly thereafter enter the Mark O. Hatfield Wilderness. The trail then ducks into the canyon of Camp Creek, crossing this small stream without the benefit of a bridge. From here you make a gradual uphill through a relatively open forest to a fine campsite at the junction with Casey Creek Trail at 4 miles. To obtain water here, you must follow a steep and unsigned 0.3-mile side trail that goes down to a scenic little mossy glen at the confluence of Herman and East Fork Herman creeks.

Go straight at the junction, staying on the Herman Creek Trail, and go gradually uphill. The forest here is mostly composed of western hemlocks, Douglas firs, and western red cedars, but there are also lots of vine maples in the understory, which add a touch of color in late October. About 0.8 mile from the Casey Creek junction, you pass below a trickling waterfall on Hazel Creek, and then cross Slide and Mullinix creeks, the latter perhaps getting your feet wet before midsummer. There is a fair campsite on the right about 100 yards before you cross Mullinix Creek.

The trail continues with its long, slow, steady ascent, always in forest and crossing several trickling creeks along the way to a junction just before spacious Cedar Swamp Camp at 7.3 miles. Situated in a grove of big, old trees, this camp is a good destination for a moderate overnight trip.

If you are continuing beyond Cedar Swamp, go straight at the junction and walk mostly on the level for 0.4 mile through a wet area crowded with devils club to a crossing of what is left of East Fork Herman Creek. The crossing is an easy ford, but if you prefer to keep your feet dry, look for a log a little upstream from the trail crossing. About 100 yards after the crossing you'll find a nice camp. The best sites are at the end of a short, unmarked spur trail that goes left toward the creek.

The trail soon resumes its steady uphill into higher-elevation forest with lots of beargrass on the forest floor. After passing through a small meadow, climb a little more to a junction at 9.2 miles with the 0.3-mile spur trail to tiny Mud Lake. Although it is marked with a very small brown sign on a tree on your left, this junction is easy to miss, so watch carefully. The lake am-

ply rewards your vigilance, with fine views of a talus slope to the southeast, a scenic grassy shoreline, and a nice campsite above the southwest shore. Look for ducks and beavers on the lake, especially in the evening and early morning.

Although Mud Lake is the recommended turnaround point, hikers looking for a more challenging trip can make a very scenic 23.3-mile loop that returns to the trailhead via the Pacific Crest Trail over Benson Plateau (see map on p. 123). Excellent side trips off this route include Wahtum Lake and Tomlike and Chinidere mountains.

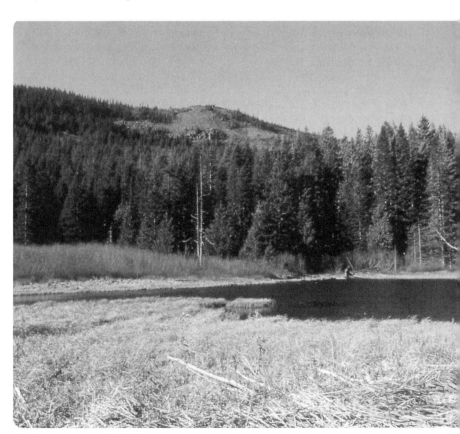

Mud Lake, Mark O. Hatfield Wildnerness

34 North, Bear, and Warren Lakes

RATINGS	Scenery **6**　Difficulty **1 to 6**　Solitude **6**
ROUND-TRIP DISTANCE	1.6 miles to North Lake; 2.6 miles to Bear Lake; 6.8 miles to Warren Lake
ELEVATION GAIN	190 feet to North Lake; 480 feet to Bear Lake; 2100 feet to Warren Lake
OPTIONAL MAPS	*Green Trails: Bonneville Dam, Hood River*
USUALLY OPEN	Mid-May to mid-November
BEST TIMES	June to October
AGENCY	Hood River Ranger District (Mount Hood National Forest)
PERMIT	None

to North
or Bear
Lakes

Highlights

These three lovely but generally un-crowded mountain lakes are all accessible from the same trailhead off an isolated gravel road southwest of Hood River. They provide a range of difficulty options, from the short and mostly level stroll to scenic North Lake, to a somewhat more difficult hike to Bear Lake, and finally a rugged hike over the view-packed shoulder of Mt. Defiance to Warren Lake. All three lakes are worth visiting, and you won't be disappointed to spend the night at any of them. Which option you choose depends on your time, abilities, and interests.

Getting There

Drive east on Interstate 84, leaving the freeway at Hood River Exit 62. Drive 1.3 miles east on Cascade Avenue, then turn right (south) on 13th Street, and stay on this main road through several turns and intersections for 3.1 miles to a four-way stop. Turn left on Tucker Road, following signs to Odell, go 2 miles, and then veer right at a junc-

tion with a sign for Parkdale. Continue another 6.5 miles, and then bear right (downhill) at a sign for Lost Lake and drive 0.2 mile to a junction on the other side of a bridge. Turn right on Punch Bowl Road, drive 0.3 mile to an intersection, and go straight, still on Punch Bowl Road. After 1.1 miles continue straight at another junction where your route turns to gravel and becomes Forest Road 2820. Proceed 8.1 miles on this bumpy but reasonably good gravel road to a T junction, turn left, and then drive 2.1 miles to the trailhead. The trail sign on your right is easy to miss, so watch carefully. There is room for about three cars to park here.

Hiking It

The trail goes south in a forest of firs and hemlocks, with an abundance of beargrass and huckleberries covering the forest floor. After just 20 yards a signboard marks where the trail splits.

To reach North Lake, turn left at the junction and gradually ascend through an open and attractive mid-elevation forest. After 0.7 mile of gentle and easy hiking, you come to a fork. Turn left on North Lake Trail, walk 25 yards, and then turn right at a second junction. In 0.1 mile this path leads to a fine camp at the south end of North Lake. This scenic pool is backed by a rockslide on the ridge that rises above the east shore and supports a healthy population of brook trout. There are additional good camps on the north and east shores.

If you are heading for either Bear or Warren Lake, turn right at the junction near the trailhead onto the Mt. Defiance Trail and make your way gently uphill through a forest of western and mountain hemlocks, Douglas firs, Pacific silver firs, and lodgepole pines. The trail's grade gradually increases as you steadily ascend to the northeast, making your way up the ridge toward Mt. Defiance. At 0.6 mile is an obvious but usually unsigned junction.

To reach Bear Lake, veer left at the junction and hike mostly on the level through an attractive and relatively open forest. At 0.4 mile from the Mt.

Defiance Trail, you pass through a small rocky area where the trail is marked with cairns, and then descend 200 feet in 0.3 mile to a comfortable campsite at the north end of scenic Bear Lake. The talus fields and rounded summit of Mt. Defiance rise above the east side of this forest-rimmed lake, providing nice views. Sadly, that view is marred by the presence of radio, microwave, and cell phone towers cluttering the summit of the peak. The shallow lake has brook trout for the angler, but the rocky bottom makes swimming rather unattractive.

The most challenging destination of the trio is Warren Lake. To reach that goal, go straight at the Bear Lake turnoff and continue climbing through forest to a prominent ridgecrest where you can look down to Bear Lake and northeast to distant Mt. Adams. The trail turns right (east) here, following the ridge and continuing its ascent, often rather steeply, to a junction in the middle of a large rockslide. If you want to visit the top of Mt. Defiance, veer

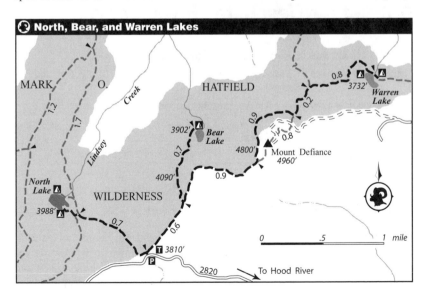

North, Bear, and Warren Lakes

right and climb 0.2 mile to the summit area with its cluster of towers and a rough dirt road.

To reach Warren Lake, go left at the junction below the summit of Mt. Defiance and gradually downhill as you round the open, rocky, west side of the peak. The views to the west are superb: Bear Lake, Green Point Mountain, and numerous other high points and landmarks of the Columbia River Gorge. Turn left at the junction on the northeast side of Mt. Defiance and wind steeply downhill through open forest for 0.2 mile to another junction. Turn right and descend partly in forest and partly on an open slope, with fine views of the basin holding Warren Lake. Upon arriving at the north shore of that lovely lake, you will discover a good campsite. Another good site lies along the east side of the lake. Much of the lakeshore is brushy, but there are plenty of places to reach the water. The swimming here is good and the scenery

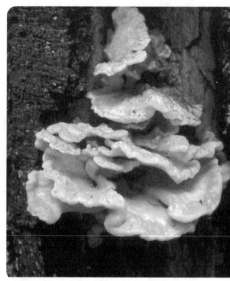

Fungus on tree beside Bear Lake, Mark O. Hatfield Wilderness

is excellent, as the lake is backed by an impressive talus slope rising above its west shore.

35 Lower Deschutes River Canyon

RATINGS	Scenery **7** Difficulty **1 to 4** Solitude **5**
ROUND-TRIP DISTANCE	5.5 miles to first campsite; 7.3 miles to Gordon Canyon, with Ferry Springs loop
ELEVATION GAIN	250 feet to first campsite; 820 feet to Gordon Canyon with Ferry Springs loop
OPTIONAL MAPS	USGS: Emerson, Wishram
USUALLY OPEN	All year
BEST TIMES	March to May / October
AGENCY	Deschutes River State Recreation Area (Oregon State Parks)
PERMIT	None. Overnight parking pass required.

Highlights

Central Oregon's Deschutes River is nationally famous among anglers who come to catch its salmon, steelhead, and record-setting rainbow trout. It is also well known to whitewater enthusiasts for its rollicking rapids and beautiful scenery. Campers, picnickers, photographers, hunters, and many others also appreciate the stream. Hikers, however, have generally overlooked this river. It is time to address this error, because this river has much to offer the pedestrian. The desert setting of north-central Oregon provides welcome sunshine to water-logged Portlanders looking to escape the clouds and mud of the west side. The steeply sloping canyon walls provide dramatic and unusual canyon scenery. Finally, wildlife is abundant and much easier to see than amid the dense forests west of the Cascades.

Although every season on the river offers something interesting—wildflowers from March to May, nesting songbirds in May and June, scarlet leaves of nonpoisonous sumac bushes in October—it is best to avoid this area in July and August when temperatures are usually over 100 degrees. All campfires must be in fire pans and dogs must be on leash along this trail.

Getting There

Go east on Interstate 84 through The Dalles, leaving the freeway at Exit 97. Drive east on State Highway 206, following signs to Deschutes River State Recreation Area, and go 3.1 miles to a junction just after the bridge over the Deschutes River. Turn right and drive 0.3 mile to the trailhead parking lot at the south end of the park's campground. A $5 per vehicle overnight parking fee is charged here. Purchase your permit at the self-service fee station near the park entrance.

Hiking It

Walk 0.1 mile south along the river to a signboard and junction at the end of a mowed grassy area. If you take the recommended loop on the return, you will come back on the Upper Trail that goes to the left. For now, go straight on the Atiyeh River Trail, which is named for Victor Atiyeh, a former governor of Oregon who worked hard to protect the lower 18 miles of the scenic Deschutes River.

The nearly level, hiker-only trail meanders lazily upstream in the narrow zone between the dense riparian vegetation near the water and the scattered sage, hackberry, and rabbitbrush of the desert. This diverse habitat supports a surprisingly abundant mix of wildlife. Look for kingfishers, great blue herons, Canada geese, minks, and river otters near the river, while animals like

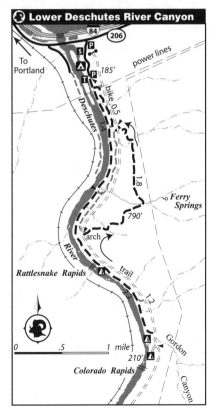

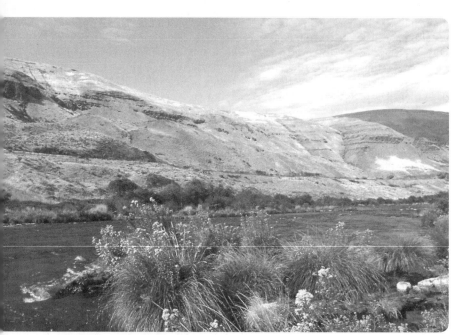

Deschutes River at Rattlesnake Rapids

coyotes, chukars, and prairie falcons can be seen on or flying above the dry canyon walls. Songbirds of all types nest in the riparian shrubs, and both rattlesnakes (watch your step!) and lizards are commonly found sunning themselves on rocks. Mule deer may be seen anywhere.

At 0.5 mile you reach a fenced tower and a junction with a connector trail that goes left to meet the Upper Trail. Go straight and hike gently up and down, still staying near the water and passing several inviting spots where you can fish, watch wildlife, or just admire the scenery. Although the trail is charming and very scenic, it is not a "wilderness" experience, since you frequently encounter signs of civilization in the form of wooden benches, power lines, and telephone wires visible on the ridge above, and trains going by on the other side of the river. In addition, a generally unseen bike trail follows the grade of an old railroad bed on the hillside on your left. The trail also passes through several fire-scarred areas, but these are natural and usually benefit grasses, wildflowers, and wildlife once the scars heal.

At 1.4 miles you go straight at a signed junction with another connector path to Upper Trail. Above this junction the River Trail is less heavily used, as it soon becomes more rocky and rough, with steep little ups and downs on the slopes above the water. About 100 yards after the trail rounds the end of a wide bend in the river, look up to the left and locate a small rock arch. Although you can't tell from this angle, this arch is just below the parallel bike trail, and you will pass right next to it on the way back. Keep an eye out as well for lizards in this area. Typical behavior for these small reptiles is to do nervous pushups while they warily eye your approach, then to rapidly scamper down between rocks when you get too close.

About 0.2 mile past the arch, you pass the roaring cascade of Rattlesnake Rapids. Just above this rapid is the first good campsite, near a pretty little rocky beach next to the river. At 3 miles an unsigned trail angles to the left toward the bike trail. Go straight on the winding trail near the river and continue to the mouth of Gordon Canyon at 3.6 miles. This side canyon presents a deep gash in the main canyon walls and supports a small creek that flows through the spring and early summer. There is a very nice camp near the river just before you reach Gordon Canyon.

Your trail angles left to meet the wide gravel bike trail/road, where you turn right (upstream) and immediately cross the intermittent creek coming out of Gordon Canyon. Just after this crossing the road splits. The main trail forks left (uphill) and heads up the Deschutes River, eventually leading to the trailhead at Macks Canyon, 23 miles from where you started. To reach the best campsites, however, bear right at the road fork, and walk 0.1 mile to a large camping area near the river, complete with a modern outhouse. Colorado Rapids rumbles along just upstream from the camp.

For variety on the return route, walk back along the bike trail, as it follows the course of an old railroad grade along a virtually level closed road. About 1.2 miles from Gordon Canyon you reach the rock arch, located a bit below the trail on the left, and a junction. The easiest way to return is to go straight on the bike trail. For better scenery, however, turn right on a possibly unsigned but obvious foot trail that steadily climbs over dry, open slopes. These slopes have fine views, and from late March to early May support a surprising array of colorful wildflowers, such as lupine, lomatium, and prairie star. After 0.5 mile you reach a view-packed high point where you enjoy fine vistas over the canyon walls and down to both the Deschutes and Columbia rivers.

The trail crosses a fence line at this viewpoint, and then contours briefly to cross the gully holding the permanent creek that flows out of nearby Ferry Springs. From here you descend gradually for 0.9 mile to a junction with the bike trail. Turn left (*up* the canyon) for 8 yards, then turn right on an unsigned foot trail that drops briefly to a junction with Upper Trail. Turn right and follow this meandering up-and-down trail past ancient sagebrush bushes that are 10 to 12 feet tall back to the junction just 0.1 mile from the trailhead. Turn right to return to your car.

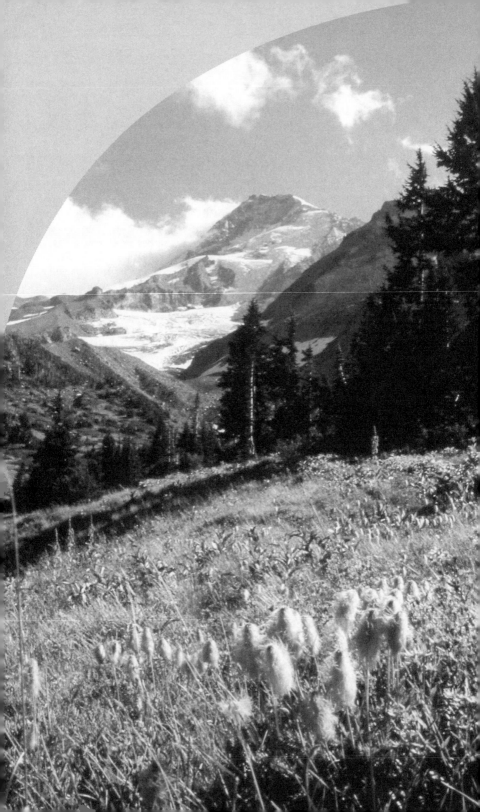

Mount Hood and Vicinity

Easily the most recognizable feature on Portland's skyline, Mt.
Hood towers 11,237 feet (plus or minus a few feet, since different
supposedly knowledgeable sources disagree) above the forest-covered
ridges of the Cascade Mountains 45 miles east of the city. Its prominent
position and considerable beauty draw outdoor lovers like a magnet,
who come to enjoy the mountain's excellent scenery, abundant wildflowers, and fine hiking trails. Backpacking on the mountain is a joy,
with all the usual alpine pleasures in almost embarrassing abundance.
The most scenic paths are those high on the mountain's slopes, but the
surrounding forests, hills, and basins hide a wealth of additional attractions worth checking out, and usually with far fewer fellow admirers
to share your wilderness experience. So, come to Mt. Hood to hike the
famous, high-elevation Timberline Trail, where the views of glaciers and
the smell of wildflowers will absolutely overwhelm you, but also come
to the Mt. Hood area to discover hidden lakes, deep river canyons, and
view-packed ridges where you may have the wilderness all to yourself.

36 Cairn Basin and Elk Cove

RATINGS	Scenery **10** Difficulty **7** Solitude **4**
ROUND-TRIP DISTANCE	8.4 miles to Cairn Basin; 13.6 miles to Elk Cove
ELEVATION GAIN	2000 feet to Cairn Basin; 2450 feet to Elk Cove
OPTIONAL MAPS	*Green Trails: Government Camp, Mount Hood*
USUALLY OPEN	Mid-July to October
BEST TIMES	Late July to mid-August
AGENCY	Hood River Ranger District (Mount Hood National Forest)
PERMIT	Required. Free at wilderness boundary. Northwest Forest Pass required.

Highlights

Mountain scenery doesn't get much better than what you find on the north side of Mt. Hood. This hike, which traverses almost the entire length of this alpine wonderland, is bound to be spectacular. Wildflowers crowd mountain meadows, creeks come tumbling down from massive glaciers, views extend to distant peaks and up to the cliffs and ramparts of Mt. Hood, and wildly scenic camps invite overnight stays. Bring your camera, pack along a flower identification guide, and savor a mountain wilderness at its finest.

Getting There

Drive U.S. Highway 26 to the town of Zigzag, about 40 miles east of Portland, and turn left (north) on East Lolo Pass Road. After 4.3 miles turn right on Forest Road 1825, follow this road for 0.7 mile, and then go straight at a junction where the main road goes right and crosses a bridge. Now on single-lane paved Road 1828, drive 5.8 miles, bear right onto gravel Road 118, and proceed 1.5 miles to the Top Spur Trailhead.

Hiking It

The heavily traveled trail slowly climbs through a forest of Douglas firs, western hemlocks, and true firs with an understory of huckleberries, Pacific rhododendrons, and various low-growing flowering plants. Look especially for bunchberry, beargrass, twisted stalk, groundsel, vanilla leaf, and pearly everlasting. At 0.6 mile you come to a junction with the Pacific Crest Trail, where you go right and 50 yards later pass a dry campsite just before a multi-way junction.

Turn left here on the Timberline Trail and make a mostly level, woodsy, 0.8-mile stroll to a junction with McGee Creek Trail and a wilderness permit station. After obtaining your free permit, go east, ascending through a forest of mountain hemlocks and subalpine firs on a root-studded trail that generally stays near the top of a small ridge, taking you toward the still unseen northwest shoulder of Mt. Hood. Finally, at 2.3 miles you break out of the forest and enter the first of several ridgetop meadows. These meadows provide great views of Muddy Fork Sandy River Canyon and Yocum Ridge to the south and straight ahead to

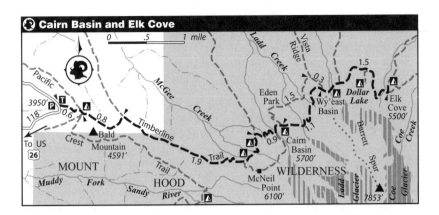

⊙ **Cairn Basin and Elk Cove**

towering Mt. Hood. Heavily crevassed Sandy Glacier covers much of this side of the peak in a mantle of ice. Wildflowers abound in these scenic meadows, including paintbrush, lupine, yarrow, aster, and wallflower, but the dominant plant is beargrass, which carpets the open areas and blooms profusely in mid-July of favorable years. There is also an unusual abundance of ground-hugging junipers in this area.

After the meadows end, the trail angles a little to the left, leaving the ridge and climbing four quick switchbacks to an extremely lush little meadow that is a riot of color in late July. In addition to the previously mentioned wildflower species, look for valerian, spiraea, avalanche lily, false hellebore, glacier lily, bistort, groundsel, and countless others. Just after the fourth switchback, you come to an unsigned junction with a use trail that goes to the right. Keep left on the Timberline Trail and wander in a daze of enchantment through lovely forests and meadows. The meadows are filled with pink heather in July and early August, which give way to goldenrod and blue gentian in late August and September. At 2.8 miles you cross a clear creek,

which tumbles in a cascading falls over moss-covered boulders.

At 3 miles you splash across a second little creek, pass a single-tent campsite on the left, and then climb a pair of short switchbacks to a small meadowy plateau with two shallow ponds. These ponds feature an abundance of wildflowers and exceptionally photogenic views of Mt. Hood. Camping is not allowed in the meadows here, but you can find some decent campsites in the forest west of the ponds.

The trail climbs to the right of the second pond and goes 200 yards to another small meadow and a junction. Go straight, still on the Timberline Trail, and hike through more of this delightful alpine terrain, now featuring excellent distant views of Mounts Rainer, Adams, and St. Helens, as well as closer looks at Barrett Spur and the steep north face of Mt. Hood. You ascend a pair of switchbacks to the top of a wooded ridge, and then come to still another meadow and a junction with a signed side trail to McNeil Point, where you go straight. A little more up and down takes you to the bridgeless but usually easy crossing of a silt-laden branch of Ladd Creek before you reach Cairn Basin at 4.2 miles. This scenic basin has an interesting old stone shelter and some excellent camps, but if you want to spend the night here, it is better to do so before mid-August, because the trickling creek that flows through this meadow usually dries up in late summer.

There is a junction at Cairn Basin. The trail to the left is a possible alternate route that goes down to the wildflower gardens of Eden Park before returning to the Timberline Trail on the Vista Ridge Trail. A more direct route, however, is to go straight on the Timberline Trail and, after 0.2 mile, come to a boulder-strewn ravine and the bridgeless crossing of Ladd Creek. By midsummer this crossing is usually a simple rock-hop, but on a hot afternoon in early summer it can be a dangerously raging torrent carrying the meltwater runoff from Ladd Glacier. As with other glacial streams, it is better to cross in the cool of the morning. If you want to use this creek for water, you should first let it sit in a pot for about 20 minutes to allow the silt to settle, and then filter and drink the water as usual.

After the crossing of Ladd Creek, you ascend a couple of switchbacks to the top of yet another wooded ridge, and then cross a few flower-choked meadows before briefly dropping to a junction with the Vista Ridge Trail in Wy'east Basin. Go straight, soon pass a faint use path that goes to the right on its way up to Barrett Spur, and then pass two mediocre camps at the east side of the basin. The lovely little creeks in this basin are lined with monkeyflower, lupine, aster, wild carrot, and a host of other colorful wildflowers.

Shortly after Wy'east Basin, go straight at a junction with Pinnacle Ridge Trail, and then go up and down for 0.4 mile to a small cairn marking the 0.2-mile side trip to Dollar Lake. Although not officially maintained, the steep path is easy to follow and the views and excellent camps beside this minuscule lake make the side trip worth the effort. Incidentally, the size of Dollar "Lake" proves what American consumers have suspected for years—the dollar just doesn't go as far as it used to.

From the Dollar Lake turnoff, the Timberline Trail goes around the end of a spur ridge, and then makes a downhill traverse into spectacular Elk Cove at 6.8 miles, one of the classic beauty spots on Mt. Hood. With a bubbling creek, acres of wildflowers, scenic tree islands, and excellent views of Mt. Hood and Coe Glacier, this place is easy to love. Please don't be a part of loving it to death, however, by camping in the fragile meadows. Camping and fires are prohibited in the tree islands of the Cove. Instead, set up your tent at one of the designated sites along the Elk Cove Trail, which drops to the left at a junction 100 yards after you cross the creek. Unless you are continuing around the mountain, Elk Cove is the place to spend the night before heading back the way you came.

37 Ramona Falls and Yocum Ridge

RATINGS	Scenery **9** Difficulty **4 to 9** Solitude **5**
ROUND-TRIP DISTANCE	7 miles for Ramona Falls loop; 18.6 miles to Yocum Ridge
ELEVATION GAIN	1100 feet for Ramona Falls loop; 4500 feet to Yocum Ridge
OPTIONAL MAPS	*Green Trails: Government Camp, Mount Hood*
USUALLY OPEN	Late April to November for Ramona Falls; Late July to mid-October for Yocum Ridge
BEST TIMES	Any time it's open
AGENCY	Zigzag Ranger District (Mount Hood National Forest)
PERMIT	Required. Free at the trailhead. Northwest Forest Pass required.

to Ramona
Falls

Highlights

Yocum Ridge, an alpine wonderland that extends west from the slopes of Mt. Hood, enjoys an unequaled position in the long list of scenic treasures around Oregon's highest peak. The views are absolutely incredible, not only of the towering mountain, but of huge glaciers, distant peaks, and even (with binoculars) the buildings of downtown Portland. Wildflowers grow in incredible abundance, adding color and an intoxicating aroma to the gentle breezes that waft over the ridge. It is a land of excitement and great scenic beauty, but rather difficult to reach. The trail here gains over 4000 feet, so hikers must be prepared to sweat to enjoy the ridge's many rewards. Those with less energy can settle for the much easier loop to extremely popular Ramona Falls, which offers few flowers and no mountain views, but boasts one of the most beautiful veil-like waterfalls in the Pacific Northwest.

Getting There

Drive U.S. Highway 26 to the town of Zigzag, about 40 miles east of Portland, and turn left (north) on East Lolo Pass Road. After 4.3 miles, turn right on paved Forest Road 1825, and drive 0.7 mile to a junction. Turn right, immediately cross a bridge, and drive 0.9 mile to a fork. Bear left, still on Road 1825, go 1.5 miles, and then bear left at a junction and quickly arrive at the large parking area for the Ramona Falls Trail.

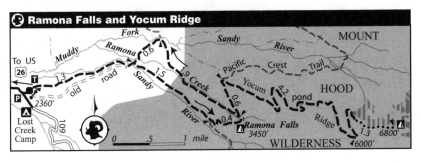

Hiking It

The sandy trail departs from the northeast end of the parking lot and travels up the wide valley of the Sandy River. After 0.6 mile, the trail meets a closed road and parallels it all the way to an abandoned upper trailhead. You then cross the Sandy River on a metal bridge and walk 100 yards to a junction at the start of the Ramona Falls Loop. For the shorter approach, turn right and walk an up-and-down path through the wide and rather desolate glacial valley of the Sandy River.

At 2.8 miles is a junction with the Pacific Crest Trail (PCT), where you bear left, make two quick switchbacks, and go 0.4 mile through open forest to a designated camping area on the right. If you are spending the night, do so here, because camping and fires are prohibited within 500 feet of the falls. Just beyond the camping area is lovely Ramona Falls, which cascades over a basalt cliff in an impressive veil of water. Immediately after crossing a bridge just below the falls you come to a junction. If you are doing the Ramona

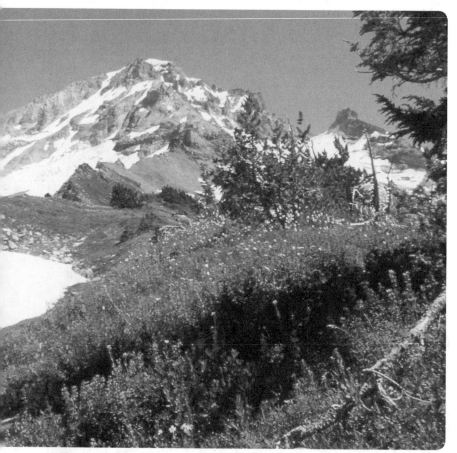

Mount Hood from Yocum Ridge

Falls Loop, go straight, and gradually descend beside clear Ramona Creek for 1.9 miles to a junction. Turn left and walk 0.6 mile through open forest back to the close of the loop at the bridge over the Sandy River.

Those headed for Yocum Ridge should bear right (uphill) at the junction beside Ramona Falls, and follow the PCT as it goes gradually uphill beneath dripping, moss- and fern-covered cliffs. At the top of the ridge, you meet the Yocum Ridge Trail and turn right.

This path goes up the south side of the wooded ridge, often traveling through jungles of Pacific rhododendron, where spiders put up thousands of webs for the first hiker of the day to break through. You pass a rocky slope and then switchback up to the wide summit of the ridge. Another long switchback, this one with occasional steeper sections, takes you past a tiny shallow pond, after which the forest gradually becomes more open and the meadows more attractive as you continue gaining elevation. In early summer, the meadows here come alive with masses of yellow glacier lilies and white avalanche lilies.

All around you now is some of the most beautiful country in Oregon. The trail passes through gorgeous sloping meadows with scattered subalpine firs and mountain hemlocks adding scenic contrast. Flowers abound, including bistort, columbine, beargrass, lupine, paintbrush, wallflower, larkspur, and countless others. The most awe-inspiring scenery starts at 8 miles when you come to a stunning overlook above the steep-walled Sandy River Canyon. From here you can crane your neck upward to look at the craggy ice sheet of Reid Glacier.

The main trail switchbacks to the left at this viewpoint, traveling uphill beneath a cluster of towering rock formations to the top of a ridge. From here, the trail turns right and ascends the spine of the ridge. You soon climb above timberline and wander through alpine terrain that features unrestricted views, ranging from Mt. Rainier in the north to Mt. Jefferson to the south.

The diminishing trail ends at 8.8 miles near the base of a rocky cliff. To reach the top of the cliff, simply trudge up one of the semipermanent snowfields or scramble up the steep rocks. On top is a glorious alpine plateau that you can happily explore for as long as you like. Ambitious types can follow the ridge all the way to the base of Sandy and Reid glaciers, but just sitting back and enjoying the incredible views is more than enough for most hikers. On hot afternoons, don't be surprised if you hear loud cracking sounds coming from the moving ice of the glaciers.

You can camp almost anywhere in this alpine wonderland, but keep in mind that the area is extremely fragile, so set up your tent on rocks or snow rather than atop delicate flowers and grasses. The only available water is from snowfields. Sunsets from up here are otherworldly, and you can even see the lights of Portland far below. The ridge is very exposed, so do not camp here in bad weather.

38 Burnt Lake

RATINGS	Scenery **7** Difficulty **5** Solitude **3**
ROUND-TRIP DISTANCE	5.4 miles
ELEVATION GAIN	1500 feet
OPTIONAL MAP	*Green Trails: Government Camp*
USUALLY OPEN	Late June to October
BEST TIMES	Late June to July / late August and early September
AGENCY	Zigzag Ranger District (Mount Hood National Forest)
PERMIT	Required. Free at the trailhead. Northwest Forest Pass required.

Highlights

As one of only a handful of lakes in the heavily traveled Mount Hood Wilderness, it's not surprising that Burnt Lake is popular. But even if there were hundreds of other lakes to choose from, this lovely mountain pool would probably attract crowds. Not only does this lake have a fine view of the wilderness' glacier-clad namesake attraction, it is also a nice spot for a swim or to fish for brook trout. As with other popular destinations, it is better if you visit in the middle of the week and try to get an early start.

Getting There

Drive U.S. Highway 26 to the town of Zigzag, about 40 miles east of Portland, and turn left (north) on East Lolo Pass Road. After 4.3 miles, turn right on paved Forest Road 1825, and drive 0.7 mile to a junction. Turn right, immediately cross a bridge, and drive 0.9 mile to a fork. Bear left, still on Road 1825, go 1.5 miles, and then go straight at a second fork, now on Road 109. You soon pass Lost Creek Campground, where the pavement ends, and go another 0.4 mile to an unsigned junction. Go right and stay with this narrow,

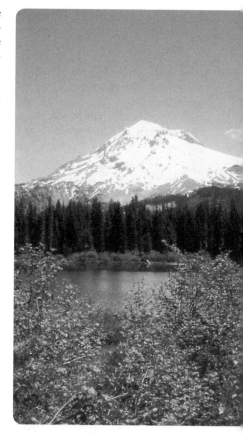

Mount Hood over Burnt Lake

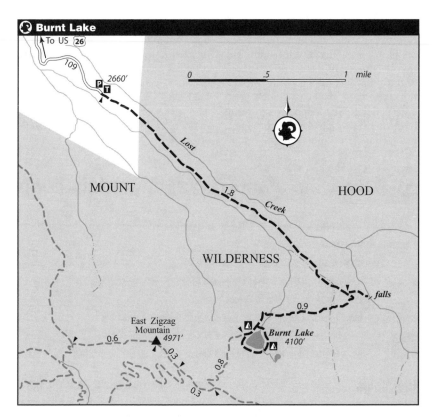

winding dirt road another 0.9 mile to the road-end Burnt Lake Trailhead.

Hiking It

The trail heads gradually uphill through a relatively open, mostly coniferous forest with only limited undergrowth. For the first 1.8 miles, the path traces a route between two parallel creeks in a narrow valley. Even though there are no views along this section, the hiking is pleasant, shady, and easy. At the end of this gentle hike, the trail crosses a small creek, and soon comes to a junction with a 0.1-mile spur trail that goes left to a small waterfall on Lost Creek.

The main trail keeps right at the junction, soon makes a switchback, and then begins a lengthy uphill traverse on a shady hillside covered with a dense canopy of firs and hemlocks. At the top of the traverse, you cross Burnt Lake's outlet creek, and soon come to the northwest shore of your destination. A sometimes brushy trail circles the 8-acre lake, passing several designated campsites along the way. Please avoid trampling the fragile shoreline vegetation by camping too close to the lake. The best camps are near the northeast shore, but the best views of Mt. Hood (and they are really outstanding) are from the lake's southwest side. The swimming is good anywhere, but it is especially excellent off a group of rocks on the lake's east shore. Campfires are prohibited within 0.5 mile of the lake.

If you are looking for a bit more exercise, consider climbing to the viewpoint atop East Zigzag Mountain. The trail departs from the southwest shore of Burnt Lake, climbing gently through forest openings, then switchbacking up a steep, north-facing slope to a ridgetop junction. Turn right, climb a little to a second junction, and then go straight and steeply ascend for 0.3 mile to the open summit of East Zigzag Mountain. A garden of tiny alpine wildflowers provides a colorful foreground for the excellent view both down to Burnt Lake and up to towering Mt. Hood. The scene easily makes the 1.4-mile one-way climb from the lake worth the effort.

39 Cast Lake and Zigzag Mountain Loop

RATINGS	Scenery **7** Difficulty **6** Solitude **6**
ROUND-TRIP DISTANCE	10.6 miles
ELEVATION GAIN	2600 feet
OPTIONAL MAP	Green Trails: Government Camp
USUALLY OPEN	Late June to October
BEST TIMES	Early to mid-July / late August and early September
AGENCY	Zigzag Ranger District (Mount Hood National Forest)
PERMIT	Required. Free at the trailhead.

Highlights

Huckleberries (delicious in late August and providing plenty of color in mid-October), beargrass (blooming profusely with tall white blossoms in mid-July), and views (especially of nearby Mt. Hood) are the main attractions of this enjoyable loop trip. Relative solitude is another bonus, because difficult road access keeps the crowds to a minimum. Although Cast Lake features no mountain views, the surrounding area is so beautiful you will have no complaints about the scenery.

Getting There

Drive U.S. Highway 26 to a poorly signed junction 1.5 miles east of Rhododendron, where you turn left (north) onto single-lane paved Forest Road 27. After 0.6 mile this narrow road makes a sharp switchback to the left and turns to rough gravel and dirt. Slowly climb this miserably rutted road for 4.6 miles, doing your best to avoid potholes and rocks along the way, to the road-end trailhead parking area.

Hiking It

The wide and gently graded trail begins as a long-abandoned jeep road that goes north from the trailhead, gradually climbing in dense forest. Throughout the summer, a wide array of forest birds will serenade your passage, including red-breasted nuthatches, mountain chickadees, golden-crowned kinglets, dark-eyed juncos, hairy woodpeckers, and various warblers and thrushes. The dense forest providing habitat for this feathered menagerie is nearly as attractive as the bird songs, featuring

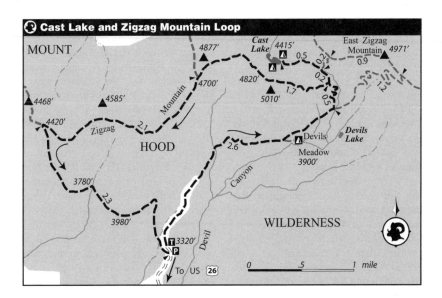

⊙ Cast Lake and Zigzag Mountain Loop

a canopy of western hemlock, western red cedars, and red alders, towering over a thick covering of Pacific rhododendrons, bracken ferns, salal, and a profusion of wildflowers. Common blossoms here include larkspur, lupine, paintbrush, beargrass, arnica, spiraea, bistort, and valerian.

At 1.8 miles the forest opens up somewhat as you go through an area of brushy meadows before coming to a trail fork. The dead-end path to the right leads to the long-abandoned Devils Meadow Campground. Keep left at the junction, now on a narrower foot trail, and gradually climb through forest on the north side of lush Devils Meadow. After crossing a trickling creek, you arrive at a junction with the Devils Tie Trail at 2.6 miles. Going straight will take you to East Zigzag Mountain and Burnt Lake (see Trip 38). For this trip, you turn left and ascend six moderately steep switchbacks through dense forest where beargrass

and huckleberries increasingly dominate the forest floor.

At 3.1 miles you come to a junction with the Zigzag Mountain Trail. The recommended return loop goes left here, but to reach the camps at Cast Lake, go straight, and walk 0.2 mile past an exceptionally pretty wildflower meadow rimmed with lodgepole pines and mountain hemlocks to a junction with the Cast Lake Trail. Turn left and gain about 150 feet in 0.3 mile before dropping to Cast Lake. This lake has no great views, but is still quite pretty, backed by a mostly forested ridge. The shore is a mix of brush and meadows, and the lake is deep enough for swimming. A rough, up-and-down angler's path circles the lake, taking you past good campsites both on a little rise above the north shore and in a grove of trees near the south shore.

For the recommended loop, return to the junction of the Devils Tie and Zigzag Mountain trails and turn right (west). This trail climbs a wide, woodsy ridge, and then traverses the north side of a nameless high point through an area filled with tangled Sitka alders. Near the west end of this traverse you enjoy your first good views down to Cast Lake and up to Mt. Hood, which rises majestically about 6 miles to the northeast. In the distance to the north you can also spot Washington's Mt. Rainier and Mt. Adams.

After rounding the unnamed peak the trail curves left, generally staying near the top of a scenic up-and-down ridge and passing through acres of huckleberries, which provide a treat for the palate in late August and a fall-color treat for the eyes in late September and early October. In mid-July this area is also justly famous for its fields of blooming beargrass. Shortly after the trail passes below a rocky high point is a junction with the Horseshoe Ridge Trail. Go left and pass through terrain that is increasingly forested, with fewer views. Nonetheless, the hiking remains fun as you go up and down for another 2 miles to a junction. Turn left on West Zigzag Mountain Trail and steadily descend a shady slope to a crossing of an intermittent creek. You then regain almost 200 feet of that recently lost elevation to the top of a broad spur ridge, before dropping moderately steeply for the next 0.8 mile. At the bottom of this descent you make an easy hop-overcrossing of a small creek, and then go uphill a final 0.1 mile to the road just 50 yards below the trailhead and your car.

40 Paradise Park

RATINGS	Scenery **7** Difficulty **5** Solitude **3**
ROUND-TRIP DISTANCE	10.1 miles
ELEVATION GAIN	2100 feet
OPTIONAL MAP	*Green Trails: Mount Hood*
USUALLY OPEN	Mid-July to October
BEST TIMES	Late July to early August
AGENCY	Zigzag Ranger District (Mount Hood National Forest)
PERMIT	Required. Free at the trailhead.

Highlights

Situated just below timberline on the gently sloping southwest side of Mt. Hood, Paradise Park is famous for its wildflowers and mountain views. The truth is that both of these features, although excellent at Paradise Park, are actually better at places like Elk Cove (Trip 36) or Yocum Ridge (Trip 37), but those locations are also harder for the average backpacker to reach. Since this hike begins at nearly 6000 feet at Timberline Lodge, your car has already done much of the elevation gain before you start the hike. Keep in mind that Paradise Park is extremely popular, so be prepared for plenty of company and try to visit in midweek or in September, after Labor Day, to avoid the worst of the crowds.

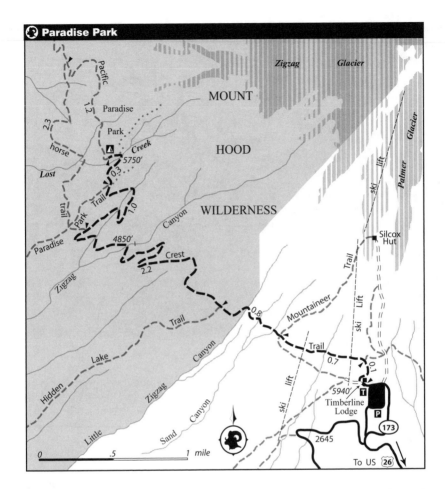

Paradise Park

Getting There

Drive U.S. Highway 26 to the junction with Timberline Lodge Road (State Highway 173) just east of Government Camp. Turn left (north), and climb this winding paved road for 5.5 miles to the historic lodge with its acres of parking.

Hiking It

From the back of Timberline Lodge, you pick up a paved footpath marked with a small sign saying TIMBERLINE TRAIL. This route climbs 0.1 mile amid midsummer wildflowers to a junction with the Pacific Crest Trail (PCT). Turn left, go under a ski lift, and then gradually wander at a slight downhill grade through open timberline meadows with good views of Mt. Jefferson and the Three Sisters in the distant to the south. Go straight at a four-way junction with the Mountaineer Trail, and soon reach the lip of the small canyon holding Little Zigzag River. The trail descends a little to this "river" (nothing more than a small creek), crosses

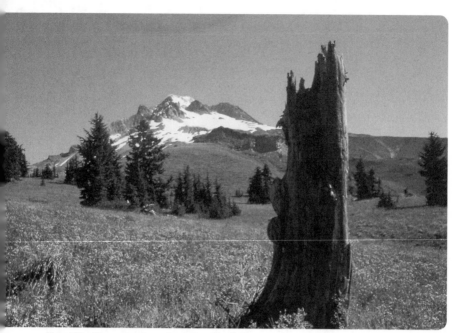

Mount Hood from meadows above Paradise Park

it on rocks, and then climbs out of the canyon. From here you travel in open subalpine forests to a junction with the little-used Hidden Lake Trail. Go straight on the PCT and gradually lose elevation, first in forest and then across open meadowy slopes where the soil is loose and sandy. After a couple of short zigs and zags, you reach a stunning viewpoint on the lip of deep Zigzag Canyon. Mt. Hood towers above the scene on your right, while below you the rocky canyon slopes plunge all the way down to the rushing waters of the river.

The path briefly follows the edge of the canyon, ducks into the trees, and then makes three long switchbacks down a cool, forested slope. There are several small creeks and springs on this segment that provide habitat for water-loving plants, including both yellow monkeyflower and pink Lewis' monkeyflower. At the bottom of the 1000-foot descent is a bridgeless crossing of the silt-laden Zigzag River. In early summer this ford can be wet and a little tricky, but by mid-August it's a fairly simple rock-hop. Less than 0.1 mile upstream from the crossing is an impressive waterfall, which is visible from the trail and can be reached by those willing to scramble over the loose rocks beside the stream. Once on the opposite bank, follow the PCT as it climbs in and out of a small tributary gully to a junction at 3.8 miles with the equestrian bypass trail around Paradise Park.

The hiker's trail goes to the right and continues uphill as you regain all of the elevation you lost in reaching the Zigzag River. At first this route ascends through trees, but then it crosses open slopes and switchbacks up a wide ravine with pleasant scenery but very little shade. Shortly after you reach the top of the canyon you reach a junction with the Paradise Park Trail. If you want to do some exploring, consider following a use trail up the flower-covered meadow slopes to your right to some fine views of Mt. Hood.

After finishing with your exploring, go northwest on the PCT to a crossing of clear Lost Creek in a gully that positively bursts with wildflowers, and soon reach the camp area at Paradise Park. Since this place is extremely popular, it is crucial that you camp only in official sites that have been used for years and can take the pounding. Fires are prohibited.

Once you've set up camp, take some time for a bit of exploring. The most rewarding option is to go cross-country around a bluff northeast of Paradise Park and wander up sloping meadows toward the rocks and glaciers on Mt. Hood's higher slopes. A somewhat easier option continues north on the PCT for 0.5 mile to some great above-timberline meadows with lots of delicate heather and views of the wide bulk of Mt. Hood's southwest flank.

41 Elk Meadows Loop

RATINGS	Scenery **7** Difficulty **4 to 7** Solitude **5**
ROUND-TRIP DISTANCE	6.6 miles to Elk Meadows; 13.7 miles as a loop
ELEVATION GAIN	1250 feet to Elk Meadows; 2700 feet as a loop
OPTIONAL MAP	*Green Trails: Mount Hood*
USUALLY OPEN	July to October
BEST TIMES	July to October
AGENCY	Hood River Ranger District (Mount Hood National Forest)
PERMIT	Required. Free at the trailhead. Northwest Forest Pass required.

to Elk Meadows

Highlights

Elk Meadows is a generally flat, grassy expanse at the headwaters of Cold Springs Creek that boasts a picture-postcard view of the east face of Mt. Hood. In midsummer the wildflower display here is quite impressive, adding greatly to the already fine scenery. As you might expect, these qualities make Elk Meadows a popular destination, so try to visit during midweek. But even if you can only visit on a weekend, the beauty is more than adequate compensation for the crowds. By turning this hike into a long loop, you can visit several additional worthwhile locations, including sliding Umbrella Falls, numerous excellent viewpoints, and some interesting treasure-hunting locations where you can look for items lost during the ski season at Mt. Hood Meadows.

Getting There

Drive U.S. Highway 26 to the junction with State Highway 35 east of

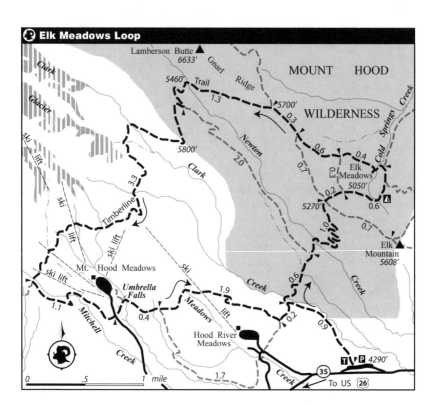

Hiking It

After a brief climb through open woods, the trail follows the banks of cascading Clark Creek, a silt-laden torrent that carries the meltwater of Clark Glacier. The fairly open forest floor here supports nice displays of lupine in July. At 0.9 mile you reach a junction and the start of the recommended loop.

You turn right at the junction, almost immediately cross Clark Creek on a footbridge, and wind your way very gradually uphill for 0.6 mile to a junction. Go straight, and soon reach

Government Camp. Go north on Highway 35 toward Hood River, drive 8.1 miles, and then turn left into the signed parking area for the Clark Creek Sno-Park.

the crossing of Newton Creek, an even larger glacial stream than Clark Creek. The trail crosses this rock-lined stream on a log, and then ascends eight long switchbacks to a four-way junction at the top of a ridge. Go straight, walk very gradually downhill for 0.2 mile, and then turn right on the Elk Meadows Perimeter Trail. As it loops through the forest bordering the south and east sides of Elk Meadows, this trail passes several campsites. You should camp at one of these, because setting up your tent in the meadow itself or the tree islands within it is prohibited.

After passing a junction with a little-used trail that goes uphill to the right, you soon reach a junction beside clear-flowing Cold Springs Creek. Turn left and walk about 100 feet to a crossing of the creek and a fork in the trail. To reach the best picnic spot, go straight and walk 150 yards to an old wooden shelter. The views from here across the waving grasses of Elk Meadows up to Mt. Hood are superb. If you eat lunch here, you should expect gray jays to come around asking for a handout (or simply stealing anything left unguarded).

To do the loop, return 150 yards to the fork and go left, back on the Perimeter Trail, as it loops around the north side of Elk Meadows to a junction. Go right and ascend in open forest for 0.6 mile to another junction where you go straight and climb along the partly forested top of scenic Gnarl Ridge. There are some decent but partially obstructed views here of Mt. Hood. At 4.6 miles is a junction with the Timberline Trail. You turn left and traverse a steep hillside as you work your way down to the crossing of Newton Creek. By late summer hikers have often placed a helpful log across this roaring stream, but, if not, you should expect a tricky and cold ford.

The trail now climbs to a junction at a minor ridgecrest, where you go straight, still on the Timberline Trail, and make your way out to a switchback atop a higher ridge with some nice views to the east. You now traverse to a crossing of Clark Creek (much easier than Newton Creek), and then begin an extended section of gradual ups and downs in open forests and small meadows. The trail goes in and out of small ravines and over minor ridges as its makes its way slowly to the south and west. After topping a somewhat taller ridge, you cross beneath several ski lifts radiating from the resort at Mt. Hood Meadows. Frequently there is good hunting here for items left behind by skiers and snowboarders in the winter.

At 9.2 miles you come to a junction in a small meadow with a nice view of Mt. Hood.

Turn left at the junction, leaving the Timberline Trail and descending through meadows and increasingly dense forests for 1.1 miles to the paved access road serving Mt. Hood Meadows. Cross the road, pick up the trail on the other side, and follow it for 0.1 mile to Umbrella Falls. This long, sloping falls is a real treat and well worth a rest stop to appreciate its charms. After crossing the creek just below the falls, the trail wanders mostly on the level for 0.3 mile to a junction. Go straight and hike gradually downhill for 1.9 miles, passing under at least one more ski lift as you enjoy occasional views down to the developed area around lush Hood River Meadows. At 12.6 miles you come to a junction. Turn left, and in 0.2 mile return to the junction at the close of the loop. Turn right and return to the trailhead.

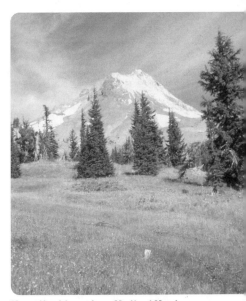

Mount Hood from above Mt. Hood Meadows

42 Salmon River Trail

RATINGS	Scenery **6** Difficulty **1 to 6** Solitude **6**
ROUND-TRIP DISTANCE	4 miles to Rolling Riffle Camp; 14.3 miles total (point-to-point)
ELEVATION GAIN	250 feet to Rolling Riffle Camp; 2700 feet total (')
OPTIONAL MAPS	*Green Trails: Government Camp, High Rock*
USUALLY OPEN	March to November to Rolling Riffle Camp; Late May to late October for entire trail
BEST TIMES	Any time it's open
AGENCY	Zigzag Ranger District (Mount Hood National Forest)
PERMIT	Required. Free at the trailhead. Northwest Forest Pass required.

to Rolling
Riffle Camp

Highlights

As the scenic highlight of the Salmon-Huckleberry Wilderness, the Salmon River Canyon has been a popular hiking destination for decades. Starting in a magnificent old-growth forest, the trail eventually climbs to the forested hillsides above the water, passes a spectacular viewpoint on an open slope, and then travels past a series of impressive, but virtually unreachable waterfalls. The upper part of the canyon is less dramatic but still very attractive,

with lovely forests and scattered spots along the river that are ideal for quiet contemplation. The biggest advantage of the upper trail is that it sees very few visitors, since dayhikers rarely travel that far.

There are several excellent camps along the river, providing options for overnight hikes of almost any length. If you are doing the entire trail, it is better to start at the upper trailhead and hike downhill. Unfortunately, even though the lower trailhead is usually acces-

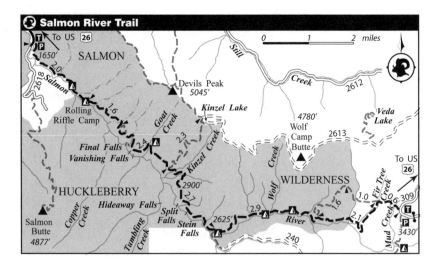

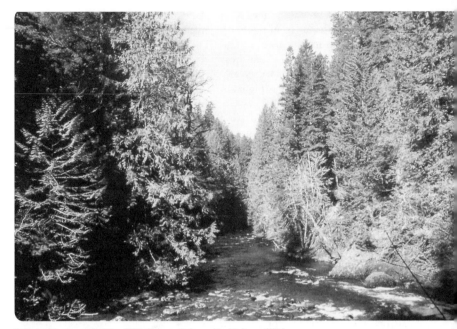

Salmon River near Rolling Riffle Camp, Salmon-Huckleberry Wilderness

sible year-round, the upper trailhead is closed by snow until at least late May. In addition, many people, especially hikers with children, prefer to start at the bottom and make a shorter hike to one of the lower campsites, instead of tackling the entire trail. To accommodate this, the trail will be described starting from the lower trailhead.

Getting There

Begin by driving U.S. Highway 26 to the town of Zigzag, about 40 miles east of Portland.

To reach the lower trailhead, turn right (south) on East Salmon River Road, which becomes Forest Road 2618, and follow this paved route for 5 miles to the large parking area on the left, just before a bridge over the Salmon River.

To reach the upper trailhead, continue 12 miles east from Zigzag on Highway 26 to a junction 1.8 miles past Government Camp. Turn right (south), following signs to Trillium Lake, and follow paved Forest Road 2656 for 1.7 miles to a junction at the southeast corner of the lake. Bear left, staying on Road 2656, and after 1.1 miles come to a fork where you bear right. The pavement ends as you continue on a good gravel road for 0.7 mile to another fork. Bear right, now on Road 309, and drive a final 2.0 miles to the trailhead.

Hiking It

The lower trail begins beside a prominent signboard and heads upstream on the Douglas fir–covered slopes above the water. After curving down to a viewpoint above a large, deep pool in the river, you wander lazily uphill through an exceptionally impressive old-growth forest of massive Douglas firs, western red cedars, and western hemlocks. Moss hangs from the limbs and covers the trunks of these old giants, while ferns and new young trees grow out of downed nurse logs. Nearly as impressive as the forest is the river, which glides along in a series of delightful glassy pools, small rapids, and quiet riffles. At 1.6 miles you pass a nice camp, and then at 2 miles reach Rolling Riffle Camp, below the trail on the right. This is a good goal for hikers with children.

Just past Rolling Riffle Camp the trail pulls away from the water and climbs steadily but not steeply up a forested hillside. You cross several small creeks along the way, so water remains plentiful even though you are now well above the river. At 3.6 miles, shortly after climbing out of a good-sized side canyon, the trail splits. For the best scenery keep right, and almost immediately leave the forest for an open slope with outstanding canyon views. The river cascades through a cliff-walled chasm almost 600 feet below, while delicate wildflowers add color to the foreground. This is the best canyon viewpoint of the trip. Unfortunately, these views are short-lived as the narrow, pebble-strewn path soon leaves the open hillside and makes a short, steep climb back up to a junction with the main trail.

Over the next 0.6 mile you pass several unsigned use paths that drop very steeply to the right. These lead to stunning overlooks down into the canyon and especially of towering Final and Frustration falls. The views are impressive but *be very careful*, because the loose rocks on these steep paths make for extremely dangerous footing and it is a very long way down to the rocks at the bottom of the canyon. People have

fallen and died from these heights, so please take these warnings seriously.

Few dayhikers go beyond this point, but backpackers can continue their journey, enjoying the solitude of the upper trail. The route stays in attractive forest nearly the entire way, always on the hillside north of the river. For the next several miles you will not see the river, nor any of the several impressive waterfalls along it. That may be frustrating, but reaching those remote falls requires dangerous scrambling and sometimes technical equipment, so don't even think about it. The trail stays mostly level until it reaches a campsite at the crossing of Goat Creek at 5.4 miles, after which you gradually ascend to a junction with the Kinzel Lake Trail.

Go straight, descend a little to cross small Kinzel Creek, and then ascend to a minor ridge crest before beginning a pattern of zigzags that go into little gullies and out to small ridges, always on the heavily forested hillside well above the Salmon River. Over the next couple of miles the trail gradually works closer to the river, until it finally comes to a fork at 8.7 miles. To visit the river, bear right on the Linney Creek Trail and walk 50 yards downhill to the water. There used to be a bridge across the river here, but it is now gone. An excellent campsite beneath some large cedar and fir trees is located just upstream from the old crossing, on your side of the river.

To continue your upstream tour, return to the main trail and soon climb away from the river onto the steep slopes above. The trail then descends once again, reaching a fine campsite just before you splash across small Wolf Creek. Another 0.6 mile of mostly gentle walking takes you to a final excellent campsite right beside the river.

The trail continues going gradually upstream, generally through viewless but attractive forest. The river remains unseen in the canyon on your right, but its "river music" is constantly heard. Go straight at an unsigned and easy-to-miss junction with an old trail that goes steeply uphill to the left, and then go up and down through forest and past the base of a large talus slope to the crossings of several small creeks, the last of which is Fir Tree Creek.

The trail now makes a long uphill switchback on an increasingly open slope with nice views across the for-ested Salmon River Canyon. At the top of the climb you cross Fir Tree Creek again, just above a small marsh, and then go gradually uphill to a junction with Dry Lake Trail, which is still signed, even though it is now officially abandoned. Turn right, immediately cross Fir Tree Creek a final time, and then climb through forest over a little ridge and down to a log footbridge over misnamed Mud Creek. From here a short but rather steep uphill takes you to the upper trailhead and the end of your hike.

43 Veda Lake

RATINGS	Scenery **5** Difficulty **3** Solitude **8**
ROUND-TRIP DISTANCE	2.8 miles
ELEVATION GAIN	750 feet
OPTIONAL MAPS	*Green Trails: Government Camp, High Rock*
USUALLY OPEN	Mid-June to October
BEST TIMES	July / late August
AGENCY	Zigzag Ranger District (Mount Hood National Forest)
PERMIT	None

Highlights

In 1917, two local outdoorsmen named Vern Rogers and Dave Donaldson packed in a load of trout to a small, unnamed lake south of Government Camp, probably hoping to create a private fishing hole. Much to their surprise, their efforts garnered them a sort of immortality, because to honor their achievement, the local forest ranger named the lake by combining the first two letters of each man's first name. The offspring of the original fish can still be caught today. On the way to the lake's shores, hikers can also enjoy fine views of nearby Mt. Hood. All in all, this short hike is well worth having to endure the lousy road access to the trailhead.

Getting There

Drive U.S. Highway 26 to a junction about 0.7 mile east of Government Camp, and then turn south on the road to Still Creek Campground. Proceed 0.7 mile through the campground, and then keep straight at a junction where the campground loop road goes left.

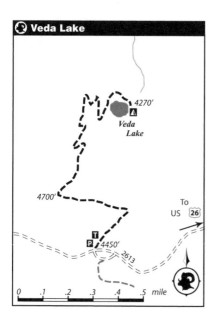

later, you reach an excellent viewpoint of Mt. Hood, nicely framed by the forested valley of Still Creek and with round Veda Lake sparkling in the basin below.

You switchback down past three more good viewpoints, each occupying an opening in the forest where plentiful sunshine allows for fine displays of July wildflowers such as lupine, paintbrush, beargrass, arnica, and showy Washington lily. The final descent is made in one long switchback across a partly forested hillside to a nice campsite on the north shore of three-acre Veda Lake. Ever since Vern and Dave stocked this lake, it has produced catchable brook trout. If fishing isn't your goal, the lake is also a good place to swim, or just relax and enjoy a peaceful mountain setting.

Following signs for Trillium Lake, drive south on a pothole-plagued gravel road for 0.4 mile to a junction where you turn right onto East Chimney Rock Road. This road goes past several private cabins for 0.4 mile to a four-way junction. Go straight on Forest Road 2613 and *slow down,* because this soon becomes a miserably rutted and bumpy dirt road. After 3.7 carefully negotiated miles, pull into a poorly marked parking area on the left, just opposite the trailhead.

Hiking It

The trail starts on the north side of the road next to a small brown sign, climbing through a forest of Pacific silver fir and mountain hemlock. Tall red huckleberry bushes crowd the forest floor, providing a treat for the taste buds when the berries ripen in late August. After gaining about 250 feet, you top a viewless ridge, and then begin a gradual descent. About 200 yards

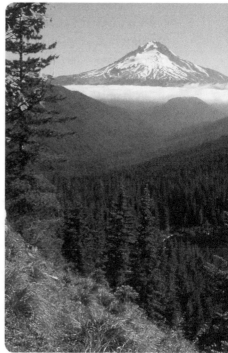

Mount Hood from trail above Veda Lake

44 Twin Lakes Loop

RATINGS	Scenery **5** Difficulty **2 to 4** Solitude **4**
ROUND-TRIP DISTANCE	4 miles to Lower Twin Lake; 9 miles for the loop
ELEVATION GAIN	700 feet to Lower Twin Lake; 1500 feet for the loop
OPTIONAL MAPS	*Green Trails: Mount Hood, Mount Wilson*
USUALLY OPEN	June to October
BEST TIMES	Mid- to late August
AGENCY	Zigzag Ranger District (Mount Hood National Forest)
PERMIT	None. Northwest Forest Pass required.

Highlights

Two sparkling lakes with easy trail access, pretty settings beneath forested ridges, plenty of fish, good swimming, and fine camps are the destination of this pleasant overnighter. The lakes are popular, so midweek is better, but they are worth a visit at any time. Upper Twin Lake is less crowded, so camp there if you prefer solitude. By adding a loop through the scenic country north of the lakes, you can enjoy some excellent viewpoints of Mt. Hood and less crowded hiking.

Getting There

Drive to the junction of U.S. Highway 26 and State Highway 35 east of Government Camp, go 6 miles southeast on Highway 26 (toward Bend), and then turn left into the large Frog Lake Sno-Park and Trailhead at Wapinitia Pass.

Hiking It

Pick up a signed spur trail at the north end of the parking lot and walk a few feet to a junction with the Pacific Crest Trail (PCT). Turn right on the PCT and, after 120 yards, go straight at the junction with a trail that heads right

(south) to the busy car campground at Frog Lake. The gently graded PCT climbs gradually in one long switchback on a hillside covered with mountain hemlocks and firs. The forest floor is covered with dense thickets of huckleberries, which ripen nicely in late August.

At 1.3 miles is a trail junction at the start of the recommended loop. Leave the PCT here and turn right, following a path that soon crosses a saddle and makes a gradual descent toward Lower Twin Lake, which is visible through the trees on the right. Just after crossing the often-dry inlet creek, a signed trail drops to the right and leads to a spacious camping area at the north end of the lake. The green-tinged 15-acre lake has pleasant views of forested Frog Lakes Buttes to the south and is very deep, so it is excellent for swimming. A fisherman's path goes around the lake, while the trail to Frog Lake Buttes climbs away from the lake's east shore.

To reach Upper Twin Lake, which features a partial view of Mt. Hood, return to the main trail and turn right. This trail soon rounds a ridge, and then climbs two well-graded switchbacks to the shallow upper lake. This lake

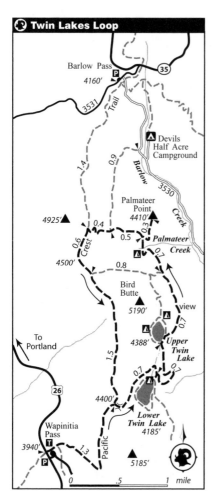

Twin Lakes Loop

Barlow Pass
4160'
35
3531
Trail
Devils
Half Acre
Campground
0.9
Barlow
3530
Creek
Palmateer
Point
4410'
4925'
0.4
0.3
0.6
Crest
0.5
Palmateer
Creek
0.8
4500'
Bird
Butte
5190'
view
4388'
0.7
To
Portland
1.5
Upper
Twin
Lake
0.7
0.7
26
4400'
Lower
Twin Lake
4185'
Wapinitia
Pass
Pacific
3940'
1.3
5185'
0   .5   1   mile

also has a shoreline trail, with the best camps above the northeast and west shores.

Since the views from both of the Twin Lakes are limited, you can hike a loop that takes you past two excellent viewpoints. To follow it, turn right (northeast) onto the Palmateer View Trail from the east shore of Upper Twin Lake and hike 0.4 mile to an unmarked viewpoint atop a rock outcropping just a few feet to the right of the trail. From here you enjoy an outstanding view of the Barlow Creek Valley and Mt. Hood. The trail continues north from here, passing a junction after another 0.3 mile, and then descending to a campsite at the crossing of small Palmateer Creek. Although it is less scenic than the camps at the Twin Lakes, this site provides considerably more solitude.

Shortly beyond the crossing of Palmateer Creek, you come to a signed junction with the 0.3-mile spur trail to Palmateer Point. This is worth a visit, even though the view is not as good as the trailside one above Upper Twin Lake.

To complete the recommended loop, take the trail going east from the Palmateer Point turnoff and hike mostly uphill through an unusually varied and interesting forest for 0.9 mile, passing one easily-missed junction along the way, to a junction with the PCT. Turn left (south) and hike gradually up and down through forest for 1.5 miles back to the junction with the trail to Lower Twin Lake and the close of the loop. Go straight to return to the trailhead.

45 Boulder Lake

RATINGS	Scenery **6** Difficulty **1 to 3** Solitude **7**
ROUND-TRIP DISTANCE	0.6 mile to lake; 4 miles with side trip to Bonney Meadows
ELEVATION GAIN	200 feet to lake; 950 feet to Bonney Meadows
OPTIONAL MAP	*Green Trails*: Mount Hood
USUALLY OPEN	Late June to October
BEST TIMES	July (for the best wildflowers in Bonney Meadows)
AGENCY	Barlow Ranger District (Mount Hood National Forest)
PERMIT	None

Highlights

There are two approach trails to Boulder Lake, a scenic pool set beneath a line of impressive cliffs and talus slopes in a small roadless area southeast of Mt. Hood. Most hikers start from Bonney Meadows and descend from this wildflower haven to the shores of the lake. The downside to this plan is that the approach road is awful and the hike, while scenic, requires plenty of uphill on the return trip. What relatively few people realize is that there is another option that is very short, never crowded, suitable for backpackers of any age, and that has a good gravel access road. The recommended itinerary, therefore, is to take the shorter trail, saving wear and tear on both your car and your knees, then set up camp at Boulder Lake and make the trip to Bonney Meadows as a scenic dayhike.

Getting There

Drive U.S. Highway 26 to the junction with State Highway 35 east of Government Camp, then take Highway 35 (toward Hood River), another 4.5 miles to a junction with paved Forest Road 48. Turn right, following signs to Wamic, and drive 14.4 miles to a junc-tion. Turn left on one-lane paved Road 4880, following signs to Boulder Lake Trail, and proceed 1.6 miles to a fork. Veer right, still on Road 4880, which is now gravel, and drive another 4.2 miles to reach the trailhead pullout on the left.

Hiking It

The trail goes west, steadily climbing through a forest of mixed conifers beside a tiny seasonal creek. After 0.2 mile you pass shallow Spinning Lake, actually little more than a pond, and 0.1 mile later reach a junction beside the east shore of much larger and prettier Boulder Lake. There are two nice campsites near this junction, each with its own picnic table. In addition to its fine scenery, the 11-acre lake supports a healthy population of small brook trout and a few larger rainbow trout.

To reach the beautiful rolling expanse of Bonney Meadows, take the trail that goes north along the east shore of Boulder Lake, and follow it up a forested hillside. After 0.2 mile you pass bubbling Kane Springs, and then climb one long switchback to the top of a ridge. Here the trail levels out and goes southwest through forest for

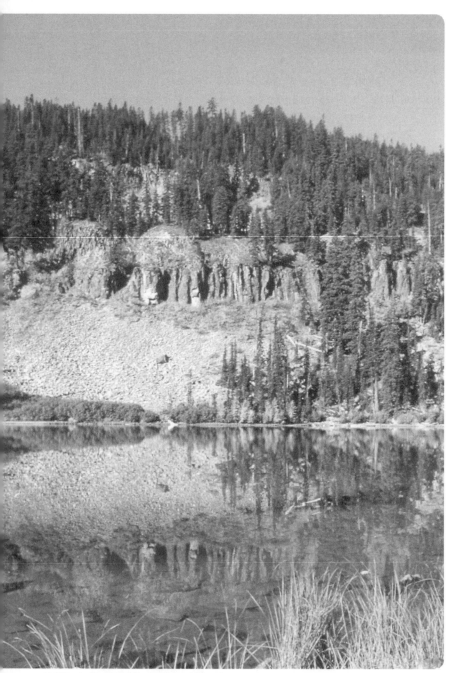

Boulder Lake, Mount Hood National Forest

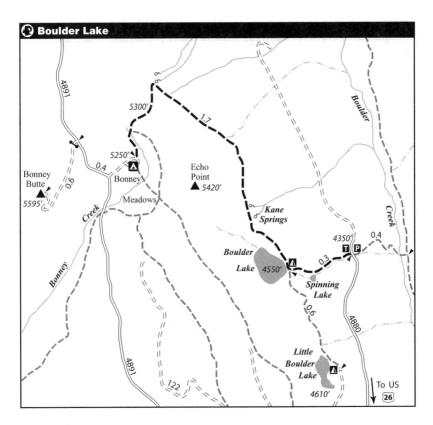

Boulder Lake

0.1 mile to a junction at the north end of the wildflower-covered expanse of Bonney Meadows. From this end of the meadow there are only limited mountain views, but it is still extremely lovely with a meandering creek, waving grasses, and plenty of wildflowers. The trail to the left loops through the forest around the edge of the meadows, while going straight will take you across a small portion of the meadows to primitive Bonney Meadows Campground, the alternate trailhead.

You can turn around at the meadows, well satisfied with your side trip, or, if you want a view, extend your side trip to Bonney Butte. To reach it, walk down the dirt access road to Bonney Meadows Campground to its junction with Road 4891, turn right, and walk uphill 0.2 mile to the junction with a gated jeep road going to the left. Turn onto this road and climb increasingly open slopes for 0.6 mile to the summit. The view of Mt. Hood from this high point makes the extra sweat worthwhile. In October, Bonney Butte is an important "hawk watch" site where migrating birds of prey are counted as they move south. Bring your binoculars and keep an eye out for golden eagles, prairie falcons, merlins, and various hawks.

46 Lookout Mountain and Oval Lake

RATINGS	Scenery **7** Difficulty **6** Solitude **7**
ROUND-TRIP DISTANCE	6.4 miles (including side trip to Palisade Point)
ELEVATION GAIN	2050 feet (including side trip)
OPTIONAL MAPS	Green Trails: Flag Point, Mount Hood
USUALLY OPEN	Late June to October
BEST TIMES	July
AGENCY	Barlow Ranger District (Mount Hood National Forest)
PERMIT	None. Northwest Forest Pass required.

Highlights

Rising like a green wall east of Mt. Hood, Surveyors Ridge is the last major outpost in the Cascade Range before those mountains slope down to the arid grasslands of north-central Oregon. The highest point along that ridge is Lookout Mountain, and, not surprisingly, it provides one of the best views anywhere of Oregon's highest mountain, just 6 miles to the west.

A short trail reaches this fine viewpoint, but backpackers can turn this into a longer and more satisfying hike by going east on the Divide Trail, a scenic route that passes a string of impressive cliff-edge viewpoints, wildflower meadows, and dramatic rock outcroppings. The overnight destination is Oval Lake, a tiny but attractive pool that is almost never crowded.

Getting There

Drive Oregon Highway 35 either south from Hood River or north from its junction with U.S. Highway 26 to a junction between Mileposts 70 and 71. Turn east onto Forest Road 44, following signs to Dufur, and proceed 3.8 miles to a junction just after you top a ridge. Turn right onto gravel Road 4410, drive 4.6 miles to a junction, and then turn left to reach the signed trailhead in about 0.1 mile.

Hiking It

The well-developed trail goes south following a long-abandoned jeep road that makes a very gradual climb beside a large meadow called High Prairie. In July this meadow is a riot of wildflowers, with false hellebore, bistort, aster, valerian, dandelion, and a host of other blossoms putting on a grand display of color. After passing a small spring at 0.4 mile, you leave the meadow for a forest of subalpine firs and mountain hemlocks as the trail, or old road, gradually ascends a couple of lazy switchbacks to a ridgetop junction. Turn left on the main route and cross increasingly open and rocky slopes to a fork just below the summit of Lookout Mountain. If you want to visit the summit, simply veer left and walk uphill for the final 75 yards. The view from this old fire lookout site is outstanding, including distant snow-covered peaks from Mt. Rainier in the north to the Three Sisters in the south, east to the dry wheat fields and grasslands of eastern Oregon, and especially

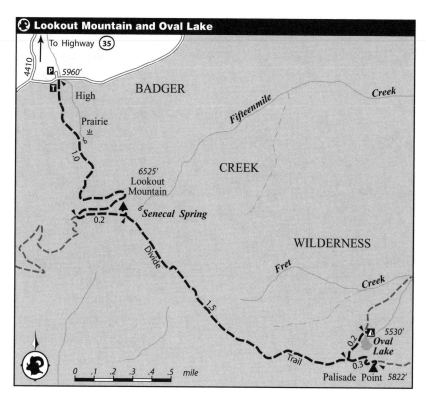

Lookout Mountain and Oval Lake

To Highway 35

4410

P 5960'

T

High

Prairie

BADGER

CREEK

WILDERNESS

Fifteenmile

Creek

6525'
Lookout
Mountain

Senecal Spring

Divide

Fret

Creek

1.0

0.2

1.5

Trail

0.2

5530'
Oval
Lake

0.3

Palisade Point 5822'

0 .1 .2 .3 .4 .5 mile

west to the towering summit of Mt. Hood. Twisted whitebark pines make interesting frames for photographs and a smattering of wildflowers add color to the scene.

To reach Oval Lake, return to the junction just below the summit and go east, leaving the old road and following the Divide Trail. This footpath steeply descends a flower-covered slope that hosts such beautiful varieties as cliff penstemon, stonecrop, buckwheat, and skyrocket gilia. Once at the bottom of this slope, the trail traces a course along a scenic ridgeline going in and out of forest, frequently passing silvery old snags and wildflower meadows along the way. At several points it is possible to follow short side trails that go right (south) to rock outcroppings with ter-

rific views to the south over Badger Lake and the Badger Creek Wilderness to distant Mt. Jefferson. The trail has at least four steep downhill segments interspersed with more gentle sections.

At 2.7 miles you reach a prominent junction. Turn left and wander downhill through a dense forest of mountain hemlocks for 0.2 mile to tiny and shallow Oval Lake. The best camps are on the other side of the outlet creek above the north shore. Although a welcome permanent source of water, this lake has only marginal swimming, since it is very shallow and rather muddy. The lake has no fish. There are some decent views looking south over the water to the crags of Palisade Point.

If you have the time and energy, it is worth taking a side trip to Palisade

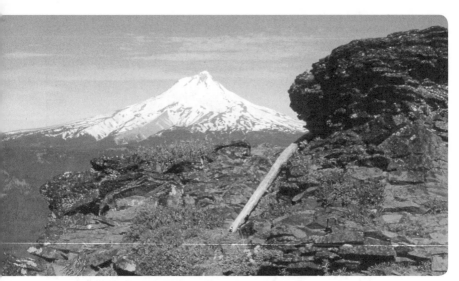

Mount Hood from Lookout Mountain, Badger Creek Wilderness

Point. To reach it, return to the Divide Trail and turn left (east), climbing a few short but steep switchbacks. After 0.3 mile, you leave the trail and walk south about 50 yards to the dramatic clifftop viewpoint atop Palisade Point. After admiring the views, especially to the south of Mt. Jefferson, return the way you came.

47 Badger Creek

RATINGS	Scenery **5** Difficulty **2** Solitude **7**
ROUND-TRIP DISTANCE	5.8 miles (with many shorter and longer options)
ELEVATION GAIN	450 feet
OPTIONAL MAP	*Green Trails: Flag Point*
USUALLY OPEN	March to November
BEST TIMES	May / late October
AGENCY	Barlow Ranger District (Mount Hood National Forest)
PERMIT	None

Highlights

Although it has none of the spectacular mountain scenery found on some of the other trails in this book, this uncrowded hike up charming Badger Creek has plenty to recommend it. The trail is easy and fun for backpackers of any age. The creek is very pretty and a constant joy to walk beside. The forest is exceptionally attractive, and due to its eastside location, it features an interesting and unusual mix of trees, shrubs, and flowers found both in the high mountains and in the dry semi-desert lands of eastern Oregon. Finally, there are dozens of possible campsites along the way, so hikers can travel whatever distance suits their abilities and interests.

Getting There

Drive U.S. Highway 26 to the junction with State Highway 35 east of Government Camp. Continue southeast on U.S. 26 for 11.1 miles, then turn left onto paved Forest Road 43, following signs to Rock Creek Reservoir. Drive 6 miles, turn right on paved Road 48, and proceed 15.5 miles to an unsigned junction just as the main road completes a sweeping turn to the right. Turn left on Road 4810, go 0.2 mile to a fork, and then bear right, still on one-lane paved Road 4810. After another 2 miles turn right on Road 4811, following signs to Bonney Crossing Campground, drive 1.3 miles, and then turn right on gravel Road 2710. Proceed 1.7 miles and come to the trailhead on the left immediately after a bridge over Badger Creek.

Hiking It

The gentle creekside trail heads upstream in an open and exceptionally attractive forest of grand firs, Douglas firs, western red cedars, ponderosa pines, and Oregon white oaks. The dappled sunshine coming through this forest provides enough light for many low shrubs, dominated by snowberry and wild rose. Along the creek are willows and other water-loving plants. The forest here is particularly beautiful in May, when the wildflowers are abundant, and in mid- to late October, when the fall colors from the oaks, Douglas maples, willows, and red alders are quite showy. Clear-flowing Badger Creek is a constant and welcome companion, adding its beauty to the mix as it tumbles joyfully over boulders in a narrow streambed on your left.

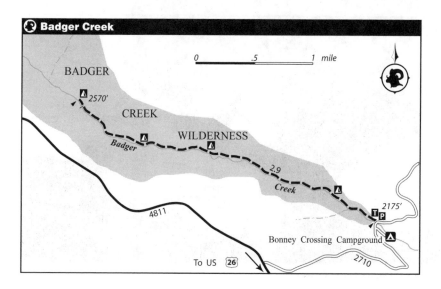

The first of many inviting campsites comes at 0.4 mile, and above that point the generally flat ground at the bottom of this steep-walled canyon ensures that you could set up camp at dozens of additional locations over the next few miles. The trail avoids most of the ups and downs that usually plague creekside paths, remaining either level or a very gentle uphill for almost its entire length. At 1.7 miles, immediately after one of the few brief downhill sections, you'll find an exceptionally nice campsite on your left. At 2.2 miles is yet another fine camp, and then at 2.9 miles you'll come to a lovely little spot where the creek chutes over a tiny waterfall between two large, moss-covered boulders into a deep wading pool. Just 30 yards past this scenic little falls is a fine campsite, the recommended spot for you to spend the night, especially if you are hiking with children.

Keep in mind that equestrian use is fairly high on this trail, so try to camp well away from the trail so horses aren't frightened by your children running around or making noise.

Hardy hikers have the option to continue upstream, as the trail follows the creek all the way to its source at artificially dammed Badger Lake, 10.7 miles from the trailhead. The creekside scenery is attractive throughout and by the time you reach Badger Lake you will have been treated to an abundance of western larch, which pepper the hillsides with gold in the latter part of October.

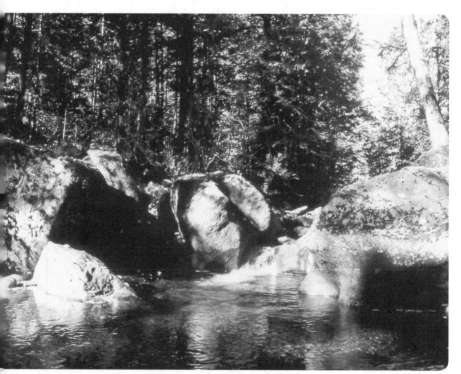

Small falls on Badger Creek

Clackamas River Country

Rising in the forested highlands of the Cascade Mountains south-east of Portland, the strikingly beautiful Clackamas River flows clear and cold through a scenic, twisting canyon cut into a contorted landscape of forest-covered ridges. There are relatively few options for backpackers to hike directly beside the river, but the surrounding mountains hide countless treasures to explore. Although there are no glacier-clad peaks, you will discover dozens of mostly small but unusually pretty mountain lakes, each surrounded by lush forests and often backed by scenic talus slopes and ridges. There are also view-packed ridges, old-growth forests, and wildflower-filled meadows all accessible by trails that generally receive only a fraction of the pedestrian traffic tramping the more famous paths around Mt. Hood or in the Columbia River Gorge. So if you are willing to forego the alpine scenery of the high volcanic peaks, the Clackamas River country has much to commend it for the weekend backpacker.

48 Memaloose Lake

RATINGS	Scenery **5** Difficulty **2** Solitude **6**
ROUND-TRIP DISTANCE	2.8 miles
ELEVATION GAIN	700 feet
OPTIONAL MAP	*Green Trails: Fish Creek Mountain*
USUALLY OPEN	June to October
BEST TIMES	June to October
AGENCY	Clackamas River Ranger District (Mount Hood National Forest)
PERMIT	None

Highlights

Memaloose Lake is a shallow gem in a scenic, mostly forested bowl beneath a rockslide on the northeast slope of South Fork Mountain. Although the hike into the lake is all uphill, it is easy enough for children, and includes plenty of things to entertain hikers of all ages. Along the way are some massive old-growth forests, a splashing creek, and plenty of seasonal berries, all ending at a pleasant lake filled with trout and roughskin newts.

Getting There

From Estacada go 9.4 miles southeast on State Highway 224, then turn right on Memaloose Road 45. Stay on Road 45 for 11.3 miles to the end of pavement and a junction. Turn right and drive a final 0.9 mile to the trailhead on the left.

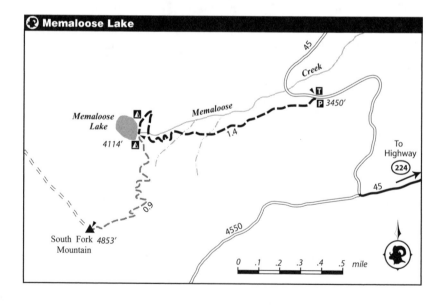

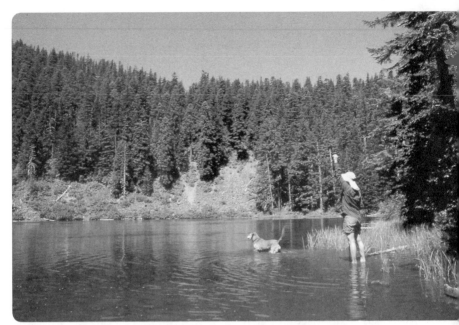

Memaloose Lake, Mount Hood National Forest

Hiking It

The gently graded trail steadily climbs the hillside above mostly unseen Memaloose Creek through an impressive old-growth forest of western hemlocks and Douglas firs. Tiny wildflowers grace the forest floor in early summer, including bunchberries, vanilla leaf, false Solomon seal, and oxalis. The path crosses a couple of seasonal side creeks, and then begins switchbacking, crossing the main flow of small Memaloose Creek twice before reaching the shore of 7-acre Memaloose Lake.

The lake holds a healthy population of small brook trout, which will interest angling adults, and thousands of roughskin newts, always a favorite of children. By late summer the water temperature is comfortable enough for swimming, although there is some mud along the shore, so you should expect to get dirty. The largest and most popular campsite is near the outlet where the trail first touches the lake, but there are a couple of additional good sites not far to the north.

Hikers who want more exercise and a nice view can extend their adventure on a moderately steep 0.9-mile trail to the old lookout site atop South Fork Mountain. The peak also has a rough road to the top, so you may have to share the view with motor vehicles, but on a clear day you can enjoy a vista that extends from Washington's Mt. Rainier to Oregon's Three Sisters. With binoculars you might even be able to pick out the skyscrapers of downtown Portland. The trail to the mountain departs from the southeast side of Memaloose Lake just south of the outlet creek.

49 High Lake

RATINGS	Scenery **6** Difficulty **7** Solitude **9**
ROUND-TRIP DISTANCE	6.6 miles
ELEVATION GAIN	2300 feet
OPTIONAL MAP	*Green Trails: Fish Creek Mountain* (new trail alignment not shown)
USUALLY OPEN	Mid-June to October
BEST TIMES	Late June to early October
AGENCY	Clackamas River Ranger District (Mount Hood National Forest)
PERMIT	None

Highlights

The once popular trail to Fish Creek Mountain and High Lake fell off the radar screens of most local hikers when the massive floods of February 1996 permanently closed the western access roads to this scenic area. In recent years, however, a group of dedicated volunteers has reopened a rugged older route that approaches this area from the east, once again allowing hikers and backpackers to enjoy the many charms of this region. And those charms are indeed many, including outstanding views, excellent wildflower displays, interesting rock formations, and a fine camp at very scenic High Lake tucked beneath the hulking east face of Fish Creek Mountain. Although it is improving over time, the new access trail is still rough, steep in places, and unsigned, so hikers must be prepared to work for their rewards.

Getting There

From Estacada, drive 22 miles southeast on State Highway 224 to the junction with Forest Road 4620 just before a bridge over the Clackamas River. Turn right, soon pass Indian Henry Campground, and drive 5.4

miles to the end of pavement. Continue on gravel another 2.7 miles and park where an unsigned road, which is blocked by large boulders, goes to the left. (If you need a landmark, this road is exactly 0.4 mile after you pass a side

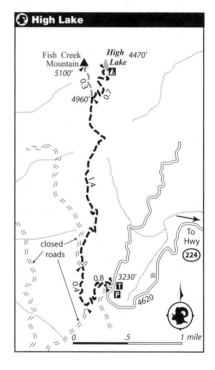

road, also going left, that is a strange reddish/pink color.)

Hiking It

The unsigned trail angles uphill to the right on the north side of the blocked road, traveling through a mixed forest of western hemlock, Douglas fir, and various deciduous trees with a thick understory of Pacific rhododendrons and a variety of smaller shrubs. After 100 yards the trail veers to the right and begins climbing, sometimes steeply, through dense forest. The trail is faint in spots (work continues to improve matters), but experienced hikers should have no trouble.

The trail makes several short switchbacks, and then tops a wooded ridge at 0.8 mile before dropping briefly to a junction with an old road. Turn right (north) on the abandoned road, which was covered with jumbles of rocks and berms after the road was closed in 1996. Grasses, shrubs, and other vegetation are rapidly taking over the surface. After 0.4 mile the road forks, where you take an obvious trail that goes up the rocky rib directly between the two forks.

The trail, which is now in good shape, generally remains near the top of the ridge using a few irregularly spaced switchbacks to gradually gain elevation. Most of the way is in forest, but occasional breaks in the tree cover open up good views of pointed Mt. Jefferson to the southwest. A few tiny meadows provide enough sunshine for late-June-blooming larkspur, columbine, arnica, and phlox to put on a nice show. Another highlight along the way is a pair of impressive rock formations that jut up from the ridgetop, hosting their own array of colorful wildflowers.

The path remains loyal to the ridgetop, sometimes ambling along

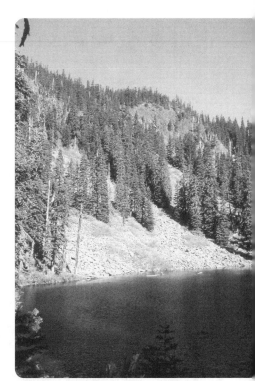

Fish Creek Mountain over High Lake, Mount Hood National Forest

with almost no elevation gain, to a junction at 2.6 miles. For a worthwhile side trip, take the trail that goes straight ahead for 0.3 mile to the old lookout site atop Fish Creek Mountain. The views here remain excellent, even though fast-growing trees are rapidly getting in the way.

To reach High Lake, turn right at the ridgetop junction and switchback downhill, losing 500 feet in 0.7 mile to the lake. This very scenic 2.5-acre pool is backed by a talus slope and features excellent views of nearby Fish Creek Mountain. Anglers can try their luck at catching brook trout, and, by late summer, swimmers will enjoy the clear 10-foot-deep water. The best campsite is above the lake's south shore.

50 Shining Lake

RATINGS	Scenery **7** Difficulty **3** Solitude **6**
ROUND-TRIP DISTANCE	8.8 miles
ELEVATION GAIN	800 feet
OPTIONAL MAPS	*Green Trails: Fish Creek Mountain, High Rock*
USUALLY OPEN	Late June to October
BEST TIMES	Late August to mid-October
AGENCY	Clackamas River Ranger District (Mount Hood National Forest)
PERMIT	None

Highlights

If your car can handle the rough road to the trailhead, the hike into Shining Lake is a relatively easy route that leads to that rarest of phenomena, a scenic mountain lake that is almost never crowded. As with most lakes in our mountains, you should expect plenty of mosquitoes in July. Due to the bugs, it is usually more enjoyable to make this hike either at huckleberry time in late August or fall-color time in October.

Getting There

Go 26 miles southeast of Estacada on Oregon Highway 224 to a junction immediately after a bridge over Oak Grove Fork Clackamas River. Turn left on paved Forest Road 57, proceed 7.5 miles, and then turn left (north) on Road 58. Stay on this single-lane paved road for 7.1 miles to a ridgetop junction, and then turn left on paved Road 4610. Drive 1.3 miles, and then, where the road makes a turn to the right, bear slightly left onto Road 240, a rocky dirt track. Slowly drive 4.3 miles on this very rough road to a fork, veer right (uphill), and then go 0.1 mile

and park in the primitive Frazier Fork Campground.

Hiking It

The trail begins as an abandoned jeep road that goes northwest from the campground. The first 0.3 mile includes several obstacles such as large boulders, holes, and berms that are designed to keep out motor vehicles while allowing access for hikers, horses, and mountain bikers. The trail stays near the top of Indian Ridge, mostly in a forest of small western and mountain hemlocks, noble firs, and Douglas firs, but with several small openings that provide fine views to the northeast of the rugged Signal Buttes and distant Mt. Hood. The entire route is lined with huckleberries (delicious in late August), as well as beargrass and Pacific rhododendrons, both of which bloom in early July. The hiking is easy, since the ridgetop route is never steep, with only gradual ups and downs.

Stay on the main route at a couple of indistinct intersections until you come to a major unsigned fork at 3.4 miles. Go right and walk 100 yards to an old campsite complete with a broken-down picnic table. To reach

Shining Lake

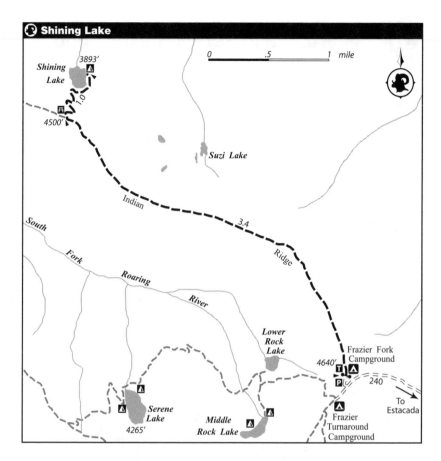

Shining Lake, look for an obvious foot trail that departs from the north side of the old campsite and follow it down a partially open north-facing slope with nice views of Mt. Hood. In 1 mile this well-graded trail uses five switchbacks to descend 600 feet to a lovely and spacious campsite above the northeast shore of 12-acre Shining Lake. This very scenic and nearly circular pool sits in an old glacial cirque, and is backed by forests and talus slopes. With beautifully clear water and a maximum depth of 24 feet, this lake is ideal for both fishing and swimming.

51 Shellrock and Serene Lakes Loop

RATINGS	Scenery **7** Difficulty **1 to 6** Solitude **4**
ROUND-TRIP DISTANCE	1.4 miles to Shellrock Lake; 6 miles to Middle Rock Lake; 12 miles as a loop
ELEVATION GAIN	200 feet to Shellrock Lake; 1250 feet to Middle Rock Lake; 2050 feet as a loop
OPTIONAL MAPS	*Green Trails: Fish Creek Mountain, High Rock*
USUALLY OPEN	Late June to October
BEST TIMES	Late August to mid-October
AGENCY	Clackamas River Ranger District (Mount Hood National Forest)
PERMIT	None

Highlights

This outstandingly scenic hike has a little of everything. Among other things, the trail passes several very scenic lakes, a wildflower-covered mountain meadow, fine high-elevation forests, viewpoints to distant snow-capped peaks, and fields of tasty huckleberries. There are three different backpacking options, so hikers can select among a very short and easy outing to scenic Shellrock Lake, a longer but still fairly easy trip to Middle Rock Lake, or a more strenuous loop past Serene Lake and Cache Meadow.

Although early summer is beautiful here, with an abundance of wildflowers, that is also when the mosquitoes outnumber the wildflowers by about 10,000 to one (at least by this author's rough estimate). Try late summer for a more enjoyable experience.

Getting There

Go 26 miles southeast of Estacada on Oregon Highway 224 to a junction immediately after a bridge over Oak Grove Fork Clackamas River. Turn left on paved Forest Road 57, proceed 7.5 miles, and then turn left (north) on Road 58. Stay on this single-lane paved road for 3.1 miles, and then turn left on gravel Road 5830. Drive this good gravel road for 5.2 miles to a junction with the turnoff to Hideaway Lake Campground, go straight and continue 0.3 mile to the signed trailhead on the right.

Hiking It

Your route goes north from the trailhead, initially gaining a little elevation, and then contouring across an open slope through a recovering clear-cut. Huckleberries and wildflowers are common here, as they are for most of this hike. After 0.5 mile you enter an old-growth forest shortly before the path takes you through a broken-down wooden gate, crosses a little creek, and comes to the south shore of Shellrock Lake. This fairly large but shallow lake is very scenic, with a talus slope to the west and surrounded by attractive forests. There are several good campsites along the east shore near the trail. The lake makes a good overnight destination for hikers with young children.

Shellrock and Serene Lakes Loop

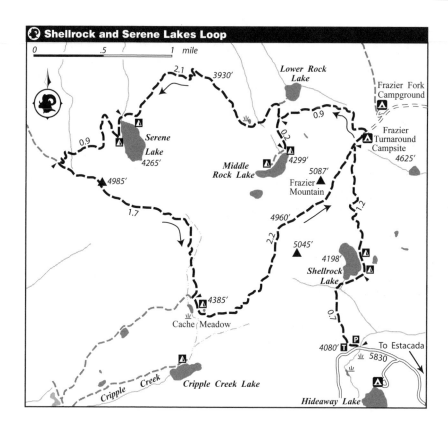

To continue the trip, hike to the northeast corner of Shellrock Lake and follow the trail as it climbs fairly steeply through forest for about 1 mile to a junction with an abandoned jeep road, now used as a trail. This junction marks the start of the recommended loop.

Turn right and descend for 200 yards to a trailhead at primitive and waterless Frazier Turnaround Campsite, which is little more than a wide spot at the end of a miserable dirt road. Pick up the continuation of the loop from the north end of the camp area, and descend in lazy turns through a lovely forest for 0.9 mile to a junction. To reach very scenic Middle Rock

Lake, turn left and hike uphill for 0.2 mile on a trail lined with tall huckleberry bushes to an excellent camp at the northwest end of this 15-acre gem. Frazier Mountain rises in impressive cliffs above the east shore of this deep lake, providing fine scenery. There is another good campsite about 0.1 mile along the west shore, reached by a brushy, unmaintained path. This lake makes a good intermediate destination if you don't want to do the full loop.

If you are tackling the entire loop, return to the main trail and go down a forested hillside for 0.1 mile to a junction with the spur trail to Lower Rock Lake, which is neither as large nor as scenic as Middle Rock Lake. Turn left,

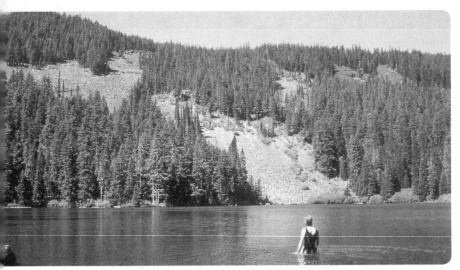

Shellrock Lake, Mount Hood National Forest

still on the main trail, soon pass a small marshy area, and then go up and down across a hillside, where you enjoy occasional views to the north over the deep canyon of Roaring River. The trail then climbs a series of short but rather steep switchbacks before going up and down once again to initially unseen Serene Lake. Unsigned use paths go left to possible campsites. After crossing the lake's outlet creek, the trail turns left and follows the shore to a large and popular camp area along the west side of this 20-acre, very deep, and invitingly swimmable lake.

The loop trail departs from this camp, climbing the forested hillside to the northwest, and then ascending a series of long switchbacks and traverses to a ridgetop junction. Turn left and continue uphill in forest for 0.3 mile on a trail that is lined with tall rhododendron bushes to a clifftop viewpoint with a fine view down to Serene Lake and northeast to distant Mt. Hood. The trail now descends, gradually at first but then rather steeply, losing

almost 600 feet before finally leveling off as it passes a narrow little meadow along a seasonal creek.

After following this creek for about 0.2 mile, you go left at a poorly signed junction and skirt Cache Meadow, where there is a permanent pond and a fine campsite. Just after the snowmelt in June this meadow comes alive with the showy white blossoms of marsh marigolds. Later in the summer, the meadow sports a mat of pink shooting stars.

Just beyond the campsite, the trail passes to the right of a seasonal pond, and then goes steeply uphill in forest for almost 1 mile before leveling out on a forested plateau. Here the route follows a long-abandoned jeep road that soon leaves the forest and crosses a rocky hillside with fine views to the south of pointed Mt. Jefferson. Shortly after the trail returns to forest, you close the loop back at the junction near Frazier Turnaround Campsite. Turn sharply right and return past Shellrock Lake the way you came.

52 Peechuck Lookout

RATINGS	Scenery **6** Difficulty **7** Solitude **8**
ROUND-TRIP DISTANCE	7.2 miles (including 1.2-mile side trip to Rooster Rock)
ELEVATION GAIN	2200 feet (including 350 feet in side trip to Rooster Rock)
OPTIONAL MAP	USGS: Rooster Rock
USUALLY OPEN	June to November
BEST TIMES	Mid- to late June
AGENCY	Salem District, Bureau of Land Management
PERMIT	None

Highlights

This hike takes you to a beautifully restored fire lookout in a little-known section of the western Cascades. The historic lookout, which is open to campers on a first-come, first-served basis, provides a cozy shelter, wooden sleeping platforms, and some wonderful views. On the downside, the trail is very steep, and you will have to carry plenty of water, since there is no convenient source near the lookout. This hike is particularly beautiful in the latter part of June when blooming

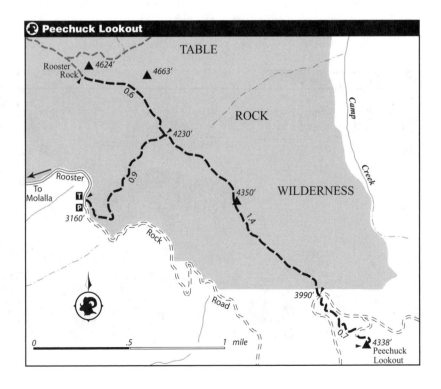

beargrass and rhododendrons bring color to the forest.

Getting There

From Exit 10 off Interstate 205 in Oregon City, go 13 miles south on State Highway 213 to the junction with Highway 211. Turn left (east), drive 2.1 miles through the town of Molalla, then turn right (south) on South Mathias Road. After 0.3 mile turn left on South Feyrer Park Road, drive 1.7 miles, and then turn right at a T junction onto South Dickey Prairie Road. Stay on this winding paved road for 5.4 miles, through several minor intersections, and then turn right at a small brown sign for MOLALLA RIVER RECREATION CORRIDOR. This single-lane paved road immediately crosses a bridge, and then follows a scenic, winding course along the river for 13.1 miles to a junction. Bear right on the main road, which immediately crosses a bridge over the Table Rock Fork Mo-lalla River and turns to gravel. After 2.2 miles bear left onto narrow Rooster Rock Road, go 1.8 miles to the Bull Creek Trailhead, then continue driving another 4.4 miles to a signed trailhead pullout on the right.

Hiking It

Walk back down the road about 15 yards from the pullout and look for an obscure trail going up the road cut to the east. The brushy trail almost immediately enters the Table Rock Wilderness, and then climbs quite steeply in a dense forest of red alders, western hemlocks, and Douglas firs, with a tangle of Pacific rhododendrons and vine maples below. The uphill abates briefly where the trail makes a turn to the left, but then becomes steep once again and remains unrelentingly so all the way to an unsigned ridgetop junction at 0.9 mile.

For an excellent side trip, turn left at this junction and walk gently uphill

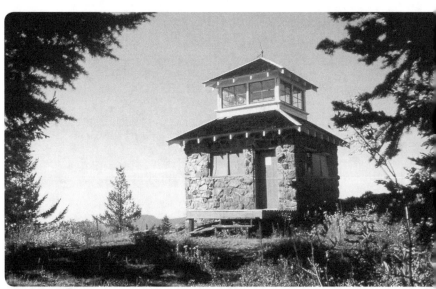

Peechuck Lookout

for 0.6 mile to Rooster Rock. For a better look at this rock's numerous jagged spires, leave the trail and scramble uphill through forest for about 150 yards to some very photogenic locations directly beneath the crags.

To reach Peechuck Lookout, go right (southeast) at the ridgetop junction and hike up and down through viewless forest as you climb over a prominent knoll, and then descend to a junction with a rough road. There is a trailhead signboard here, even though this road is gated closed to private vehicles about 5.5 miles down the hill. The sometimes sketchy trail crosses the road and ascends a series of short, steep switchbacks before coming to an abandoned jeep road. You turn up this road, follow it 50 yards to its end, and then climb a good trail for 0.2 mile to Peechuck Lookout.

Originally built in 1932, this lookout went out of service in 1964 and subsequently deteriorated. Starting in 1989, however, volunteers and Bureau of Land Management workers began to restore the structure. The historic building is now the last remaining stone lookout in Oregon and one of only a handful nationwide. Volunteers are responsible for the upkeep of the lookout and welcome overnight use, but visitors are asked to keep the lookout clean and in good condition. Trees are rapidly growing to block the view, but there continues to be a particularly good perspective of impressive Table Rock to the northwest.

53 Pansy and Twin Lakes

RATINGS	Scenery **6** Difficulty **1 to 5** Solitude **5**
ROUND-TRIP DISTANCE	2.2 miles to Pansy Lake; 13.8 miles to Twin Lakes
ELEVATION GAIN	400 feet to Pansy Lake; 2950 feet to Twin Lakes
OPTIONAL MAP	*Green Trails: Battle Ax*
USUALLY OPEN	Mid-June to early November
BEST TIMES	Late August and September
AGENCY	Clackamas River Ranger District (Mount Hood National Forest)
PERMIT	None (just sign the trail register)

to Pansy Lake

Highlights
The Bull of the Woods Wilderness protects a lovely subalpine landscape of small lakes, rolling forests, and rugged peaks and ridges far from the more famous hiking areas around Mt. Hood, Mt. Jefferson, or the Columbia River Gorge. Although not as spectacularly scenic as those better-known areas, this wilderness offers plenty of beauty, fine lakes for swimming and fishing, and a good chance for solitude. This trip takes you into the heart of this remote preserve and provides an excellent sampling of everything the wilderness has to offer.

NOTE

The trails in this description are identified by number rather than name, because almost all the signs at junctions in this wilderness use only the number without any names or destinations listed.

Getting There

From Estacada, drive 25.4 miles southeast on State Highway 224 to Ripplebrook Guard Station, and then continue 4.1 miles on the main road (now Forest Road 46) to a junction with Forest Road 63. Turn right, following signs to Bagby Hot Springs, and proceed 3.7 miles to a fork. Go straight, still on Road 63, drive 2.1 miles, and then turn right (uphill) on gravel Road 6340. Stay on the main road at several minor intersections for 8 miles to a fork, bear right onto Road 6341, and go 3.6 miles to the Pansy Lake Trailhead.

Hiking It

Trail #551 heads south through a lichen-draped forest of western hemlocks and Douglas firs, towering over the usual western Cascades understory of sword ferns, vine maples, Oregon grapes, huckleberries, Pacific rhododendrons, and various forest wildflowers. The well-graded path steadily ascends for 0.8 mile, crossing several tiny creeks along the way, to a junction with Trail #549. Go right on the main trail, which goes up and down for 0.2 mile to a poorly signed junction with the 120-yard spur trail to popular Pansy Lake. To visit or camp here, turn right and walk down the path to the scenic but marshy lake, which is backed by the steep slopes and ridges radiating off of Pansy Mountain. The best camps

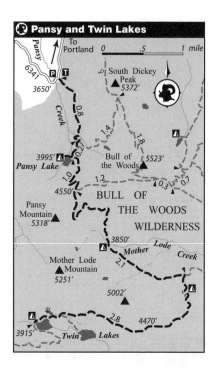

are above the northwest shore. Hikers with children will want to stop here.

If you are continuing to the Twin Lakes, bear left on the main trail at the Pansy Lake junction and make two switchbacks up rocky slopes and through open forest for 1 mile to a junction atop a wooded ridge. Go straight and descend Trail #558, mostly in forest but with occasional glimpses through the trees of pointed Mt. Jefferson to the southeast. A few irregularly spaced switchbacks take you down to a low point at a campsite beside the trickling headwaters of Mother Lode Creek. Unfortunately, this creek is often dry by late summer and cannot be relied upon for water. Beyond this campsite, it's another 1.1 miles of up and down hiking to the next junction.

Bear right (uphill) on Trail #573 and gradually climb, still in forest,

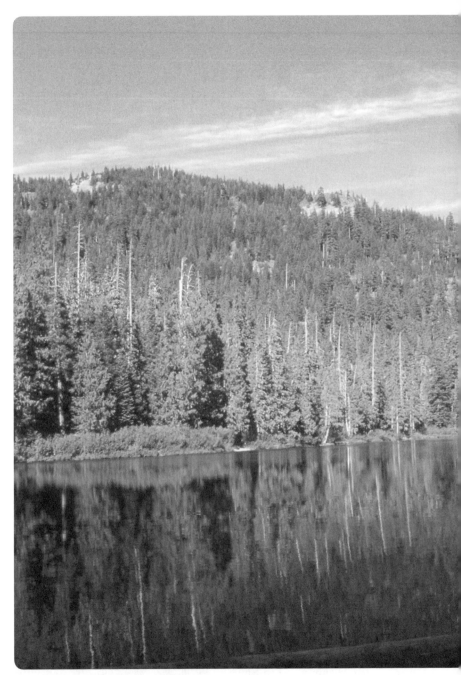

Upper Twin Lake, Bull of the Woods Wilderness

for 0.4 mile to a good and very scenic campsite on a small knoll above a pair of pretty, lily-pad-covered ponds. More climbing follows before you level off and then lose about 500 feet to the Twin Lakes, 6.6 miles from the trailhead. An unsigned but obvious side trail goes sharply left to Lower Twin Lake. To reach the upper lake, which is more scenic and has better campsites, stick with the main trail for 0.3 mile to the fine camps at that lake's west end. A rocky but delightful little swimming beach is nearby, with easy access to the deep, clear water. The lake is usually comfortable enough for swimming from about late July to mid-September.

54 Big Slide Lake

RATINGS	Scenery **7** Difficulty **5** Solitude **7**
ROUND-TRIP DISTANCE	10.8 miles
ELEVATION GAIN	2325 feet
OPTIONAL MAP	*Green Trails: Battle Ax*
USUALLY OPEN	June to November
BEST TIMES	Mid-June to late October
AGENCY	Clackamas River Ranger District (Mount Hood National Forest)
PERMIT	None (just sign the trail register)

Highlights

Nestled in a deep, mostly forested bowl, Big Slide Lake is a wonderfully scenic destination in the generally overlooked Bull of the Woods Wilderness. The approach trail is attractive throughout, with plenty of old-growth forests, a clear stream, some good viewpoints, and a pretty little marshy meadow where wildlife is common. But it's the destination that will really enchant you. With its reflections of nearby peaks, small island, fine swimming, and good fishing, this place has everything a backpacker could want from a mountain lake.

Getting There

From Estacada, drive 25.4 miles southeast on State Highway 224 to Ripplebrook Guard Station, and then continue 4.1 miles on the main road (now Forest Road 46) to a junction with Forest Road 63. Turn right, following signs to Bagby Hot Springs, and proceed 3.7 miles to a fork. Go straight, still on Road 63, drive 2.1 miles, and then turn right (uphill) on gravel Road 6340, following signs to Bull of the Woods Wilderness. Drive 2.9 miles, turn left on narrow Road 140 at a sign for Dickey Creek Trail, and go 1.6 miles to the road-end trailhead.

Hiking It

In a dense forest of Douglas fir and western hemlock, the trail begins by descending gradually for 0.1 mile along an overgrown old road. Once this abandoned road ends, the trail turns

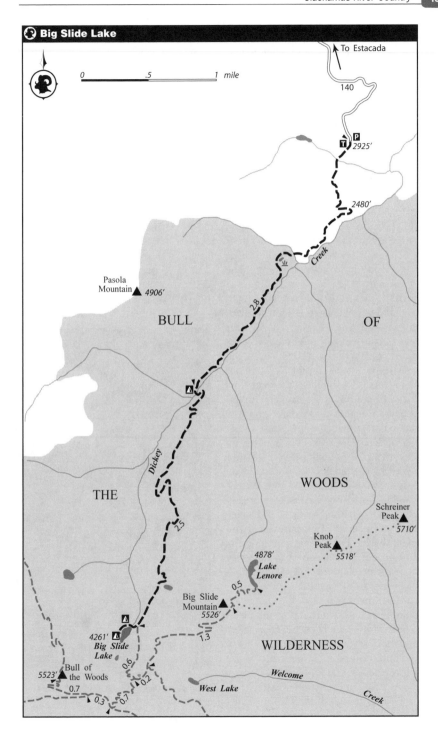

Big Slide Lake

To Estacada

0   .5   1 mile

140

2925'

2480'

Creek

Pasola
Mountain ▲ 4906'

BULL

OF

2.8

THE

Dickey

WOODS

2.5

Schreiner
Peak ▲
5710'

Knob
Peak ▲
5518'

4878'
Lake
Lenore

0.5

Big Slide
Mountain ▲
5526'

1.3

WILDERNESS

4261'
Big Slide
Lake

0.6

Welcome

Bull of
5523' ▲ the Woods

0.2

0.7

0.3   0.7

West Lake

Creek

left, crosses a ravine on a log, and then does a brief bit of up and down before winding downhill at an irregular but often steep grade into the canyon of Dickey Creek. After losing 350 feet, and shortly before reaching the creek, the trail turns right and heads up the canyon.

The forest in this canyon is very impressive, with lots of stately old-growth western hemlocks, Douglas firs, and western red cedars. Below these giants is an assortment of vine maples, Pacific rhododendrons, Pacific yews, Oregon grapes, and various other understory species, all surviving on what little light makes it through the canopy. The climb is irregular but easy, leading to a pretty little meadow at 1.4 miles, with a shallow pond that is choked with grasses and water lilies. Look for deer and beaver here, especially early in the morning. There is a nice view looking southeast over the pond to Schreiner Peak. After rounding the meadow the trail continues its irregular uphill course, reaching a pleasant campsite immediately before a bridgeless crossing of Dickey Creek at 2.8 miles. In June this crossing will get you wet, but by early to mid-July it is usually an easy rock-hop.

The trail now climbs at a steady grade, soon pulling away from Dickey Creek in a series of long traverses and switchbacks. The hillside here supports an unusual abundance of Pacific rhododendrons that are covered with pink blossoms from late June to mid-July. Most of the way is in forest, but at 4.2 miles you come to a rocky opening with a fine view of the Dickey Creek Valley and the surrounding craggy summits of Big Slide Mountain, North and South Dickey peaks, and Pasola Mountain.

At 5.3 miles, shortly after you cross a large rockslide, is an unsigned junction. The main trail goes straight (uphill), but to reach Big Slide Lake, you turn right and steeply descend 0.1 mile to an excellent campsite on the northeast shore of the 4-acre lake. This watery jewel is surrounded by forest-covered, craggy peaks; has a scenic little island; supports a population of hungry brook trout; and is the ideal depth for swimming. What more could a wilderness-loving backpacker want? Well, how about plenty of nearby exploring to such worthwhile destinations as Bull of the Woods Lookout, Schreiner Peak, and Lake Lenore? An easily followed angler's path continues 150 yards past the first campsite to another good campsite on the west shore of Big Slide Lake.

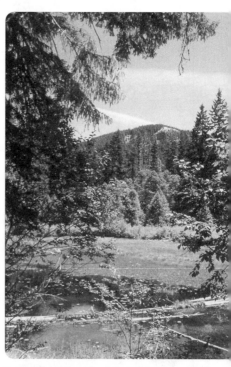

Pond along Dickey Creek Trail, Bull of the Woods Wilderness

55 Olallie Lake Scenic Area Loop

RATINGS	Scenery **7**　Difficulty **3**　Solitude **5**
ROUND-TRIP DISTANCE	9.1 miles (including side trips to Fish Lake viewpoint, Sheep Lake, and Upper Lake) with many shorter options
ELEVATION GAIN	1200 feet (including side trips)
OPTIONAL MAP	*Green Trails: Breitenbush*
USUALLY OPEN	Late June to October
BEST TIMES	Late August / early to mid-October
AGENCY	Clackamas River Ranger District (Mount Hood National Forest)
PERMIT	None

Highlights

The Olallie Lake Scenic Area is a gentle subalpine landscape full of lakes, meadows, and joyous campsites that is an ideal destination for families with children. Every lake is attractive, provides good fishing, and is a fun place for kids to splash in the water, swim, and explore. In July, the wildflowers are outstanding, but the mosquitoes will drive you to distraction, so plan to visit in either late August, when the huckleberries are ripe and the water temperature is more comfortable for swimming, or mid-October for solitude and superb fall color.

Getting There

From Estacada, drive 25.4 miles southeast on State Highway 224 to Ripplebrook Guard Station, and then continue 22.7 miles on the main road (now Forest Road 46) to a junction with Road 4690. Turn left (east), following signs to Olallie Lake, and proceed 8.3 miles on this paved then good gravel road to a T junction. Turn right on Road 4220, drive 4.7 miles, and then turn right into the Lower Lake Campground.

The trailhead is at the west end of the campground loop road.

Hiking It

The trail goes west, staying nearly level as it wanders through a forest of Pacific silver firs, lodgepole pines, western white pines, and mountain hemlocks. The forest floor is covered with grouse whortleberries, pinemat manzanitas, and the ever-present and abundant huckleberries. After less than 0.5 mile, you reach sparkling Lower Lake, a 15-acre body of water with good campsites near its northwest shore, and fine views to the east of pyramid-shaped Olallie Butte.

Near the outlet creek at the northwest corner of Lower Lake is a four-way junction. The main loop route veers slightly to the left, but for a worthwhile side trip, take the trail that goes a little to the right (not sharply right) and follow it for 0.3 mile to a fine viewpoint atop the rounded bowl holding large and deep Fish Lake. After returning to the junction beside Lower Lake, turn right (southwest) and wander uphill on an often rocky trail through open forest and huckleberry-fringed meadow

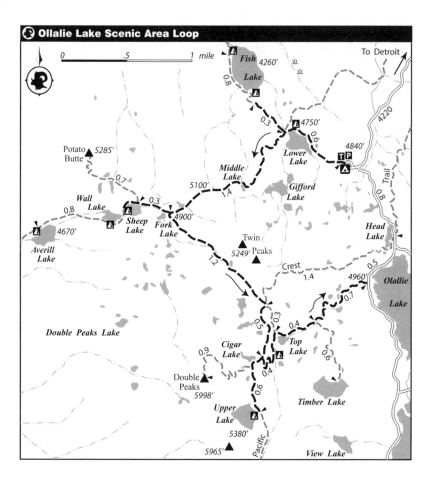

Ollalie Lake Scenic Area Loop

0   *.5*   *1 mile*

To Detroit

Fish 4260′
Lake

0.8

0.3

▲4750′

0.6

4840′
T P

4220

Potato ▲ 5285′
Butte

0.7

Middle
Lake

5100′

1.4

Lower
Lake

Gifford
Lake

Trail

0.8

Wall
Lake

0.8

0.3

4900′

Sheep
Lake

Fork
Lake

Twin
5249′ *Peaks*

Head
Lake

4670′

Averill
Lake

1.2

Crest
1.4

4960′

0.5

Olallie

Lake

0.7

Double Peaks Lake

0.9

Cigar
Lake

0.5

0.3

0.4

Top
Lake

0.6

Double ▲
Peaks
5998′

0.4

0.6

Timber Lake

Upper
Lake

5380′

5965′ ▲

Pacific

View Lake

openings. These small meadows often feature wildflowers and shallow ponds, which add to their beauty. After gaining 300 feet you come to Middle Lake, really nothing more than a pond, but which does feature a pleasant view of rugged Twin Peaks to the south.

The trail now descends to a junction at 2 miles (excluding the side trip to the Fish Lake viewpoint). Another excellent side trip begins here. To take it, go straight, soon pass shallow, meadow-rimmed Fork Lake, and come to a junction on the north shore of larger and deeper Sheep Lake. The

trail to the right goes 0.7 mile to the viewpoint atop Potato Butte (another worthwhile destination), but the recommended goal is just ahead at the west end of Sheep Lake. Here you will find a delightful campsite with a fine view of Olallie Butte to the east. For even more exploring, you can continue west on a gradually downhill trail that takes you to Wall and Averill lakes, both of which have good campsites.

Back at the junction just east of Fork Lake, turn right (south) and climb steadily for 1.2 miles past several small ponds to a four-way junction with the

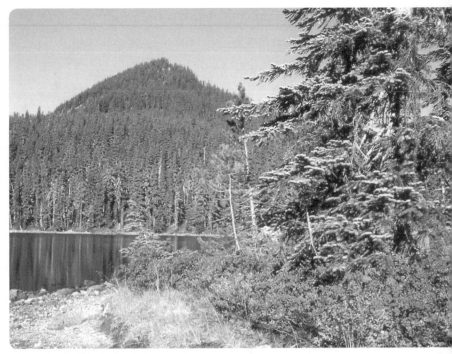

Upper Lake, Olallie Lake Scenic Area

Pacific Crest Trail (PCT). Turn right (southbound) on the PCT and, 0.5 mile later, come to a usually unsigned junction. The recommended return route goes left here, but before going that way keep right (uphill) on the PCT and almost immediately reach narrow, rock-lined Cigar Lake. This scenic lake has nice campsites and a good view of Double Peaks rising above its west shore. About 50 yards along the east shore of Cigar Lake, the PCT passes a junction with the trail up Double Peaks, which is marked only with a low cairn.

Stick with the PCT as it goes gradually uphill for 0.5 mile through pretty little meadows and open forest to Upper Lake. This extremely beautiful lake

has fine campsites along its east shore and excellent views of Double Peaks to the northwest and a scenic talus slope on Peak 5965 to the south.

To complete the loop, return to the unsigned junction just below Cigar Lake and turn right (southeast). This trail switchbacks downhill to a small meadow with an excellent campsite, and then comes to a junction at the northwest corner of Top Lake. Turn right and, 0.4 mile later, bear left at a junction with the side trail to Timber Lake, yet another good side trip. The trail ends at a gravel road beside Olallie Lake. It's an easy 1.3-mile stroll north along this road back to Lower Lake Campground and your car.

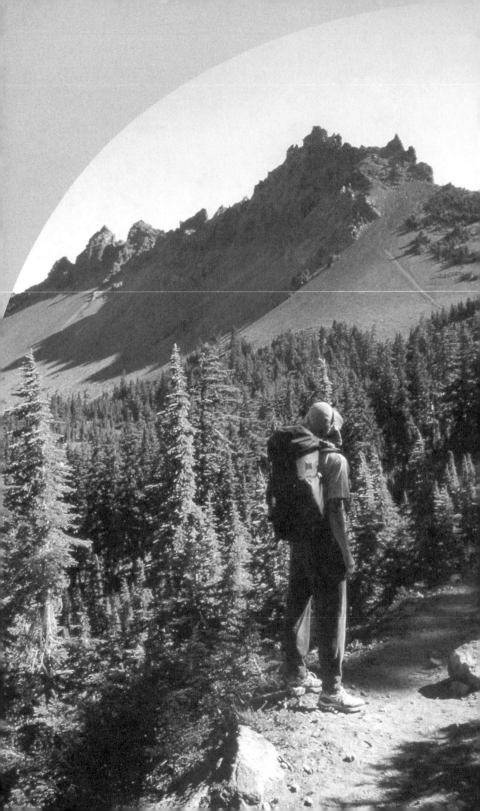

Mount Jefferson and Vicinity

There are those who convincingly argue that Oregon's second highest peak, glacier-draped Mt. Jefferson, is even more beautiful than Mt. Hood, its taller and more famous cousin to the north. Jefferson's pointed summit and changing profile from every angle support this claim, as do the dozens of lakes at its base that reflect the mountain's glory, unlike any of the tiny and less numerous ponds on the slopes of Mt. Hood. Despite being farther from major cities, the trails around Mt. Jefferson receive even higher use than those on Mt. Hood. More people means more restrictions, so be prepared for camping bans at overused locations and rules prohibiting fires in others. You even have to get advance reservations to enter certain areas. Stretching to the south of Mt. Jefferson is a somewhat less visited wilderness with plenty of attractions in its own right, especially Three Fingered Jack, the scenic remnants of an old volcano. For even more solitude, go a bit farther south to Mt. Washington, a pointed spire that presides over a little-visited but scenic land of lava and forests.

56 Pyramid Lake

RATINGS	Scenery **7** Difficulty **5** Solitude **9**
ROUND-TRIP DISTANCE	4.4 miles
ELEVATION GAIN	900 feet
OPTIONAL MAP	*Green Trails: Breitenbush*
USUALLY OPEN	Late June to October
BEST TIMES	Early to mid-October
AGENCY	Clackamas River Ranger District (Mount Hood National Forest)
PERMIT	Required. Free at the trailhead. Northwest Forest Pass required.

Highlights

Pyramid Lake, which is tucked neatly in an isolated basin on the northern edge of the Mount Jefferson Wilderness, has everything a hiker could want in a mountain lake. Although there is no view of the wilderness's namesake mountain, you'll enjoy a wonderful perspective of Pyramid Butte, a local landmark that rises impressively above the lake's east shore. And if views aren't enough, you can feast on huckleberries, cool off with a refreshing swim, or try to catch a few of the lake's tasty brook trout.

Since getting here requires cross-country travel, it is likely that even on a crowded summer weekend you will have the place all to yourself. As with many other destinations in this area, the mosquitoes can be awful in July and early August. Plan to visit in mid-October to catch the excellent displays of fall colors. The fishing is better then as well.

Getting There

From Salem, drive 50 miles east on State Highway 22 to a junction immediately after a bridge over an arm of Detroit Reservoir, and just before you

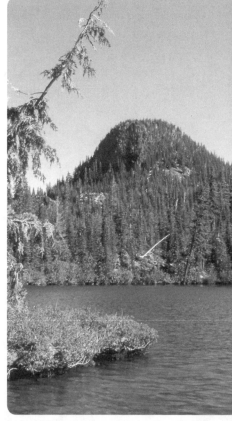

Pyramid Butte over Pyramid Lake, Mount Jefferson Wilderness

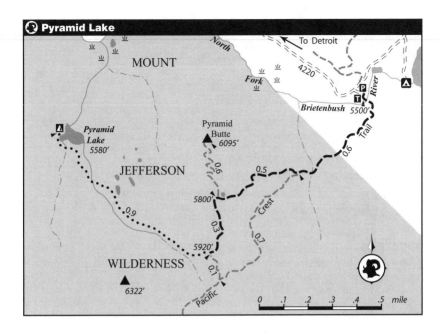

Pyramid Lake

North Fork

To Detroit

4220

P T *River*

Brietenbush 5500'

0.6

Trail

MOUNT

Pyramid
▲ Butte
6095'

Pyramid
Lake
5580'

JEFFERSON

0.6 0.5

5800'

Crest

0.9

0.3

0.7

5920'

WILDERNESS

0.1

▲
6322'

Pacific

0 .1 .2 .3 .4 .5 mile

---

enter the small town of Detroit. Turn left (northeast) on paved Forest Road 46, following signs to Breitenbush, and drive 16.9 miles to a ridgetop junction with Road 4220. Turn right (east) and drive 1 mile to a gate, where the gravel road changes to dirt. From here, the road is bumpy and rough, but it remains passable if you drive slowly. The signed trailhead is on the right, 5.5 miles from the gate.

Hiking It

The Pacific Crest Trail winds its way south, going gently uphill through a delightful subalpine landscape of meadows filled with heather and huckleberries and open forest dominated by mountain hemlocks. To the west you can see prominent Pyramid Butte.

At 0.6 mile, just after you cross a dilapidated wooden bridge over a rocky gully, is an unsigned fork. Bear right and follow a winding, up-and-down old trail that travels through forest and meadows for 0.5 mile to a junction beside a shallow seasonal pond. The trail to the right switchbacks up to the top of Pyramid Butte, and is a worthwhile side trip for those wishing to obtain a view of Mt. Jefferson.

To reach Pyramid Lake, turn left at the junction and gradually climb for 0.3 mile. Just as things start to become noticeably steeper, leave the trail and go cross-country to the right (west). Although off-trail, the hiking is relatively easy through open forest and small meadows. After about 150 yards you come to a gully holding a usually flowing little creek. Follow this creek downstream for 0.8 mile, skirting or fighting through occasional brushy areas, to very scenic 5-acre Pyramid Lake. There is a sketchy boot path that leads to the west shore, where you will find a good campsite with an excellent view of bulky Pyramid Butte.

57 Firecamp Lakes

RATINGS	Scenery **6** Difficulty **2** Solitude **4**
ROUND-TRIP DISTANCE	2.4 miles to Crown Lake
ELEVATION GAIN	640 feet
OPTIONAL MAP	*Green Trails: Breitenbush*
USUALLY OPEN	Mid-June to October
BEST TIMES	July (for the best flowers, but expect bugs)
AGENCY	Detroit Ranger District (Willamette National Forest)
PERMIT	Required. Free at the trailhead.

Highlights

Three sparkling lakes, surrounded by forest and with partial views of a glacier-clad volcano, are the destination of this easy and enjoyable trip.

Although the lakes are fairly popular, they are not as crowded as some other destinations in the Mount Jefferson Wilderness. In fact, if you spend the night at the more secluded camps at

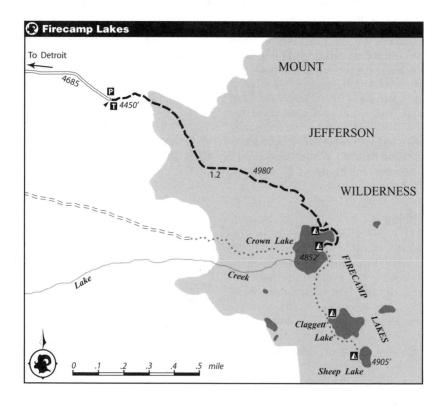

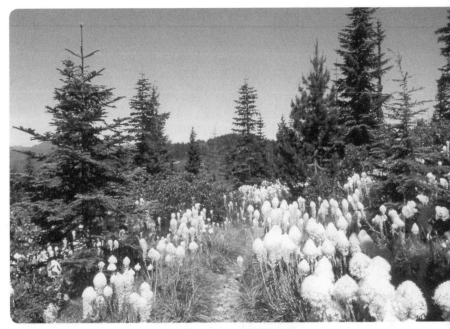

Beargrass along trail to Firecamp Lakes, Mount Jefferson Wilderness

Sheep Lake or Claggett Lake, you may have things all to yourself. In late June and early July of favorable years, the show of blooming beargrass along the lower trail is quite impressive. Sadly, mosquitoes can be a significant problem at that time, so you have to decide if it is worth it. By mid-August the lakes are nearly bug free.

Getting There

From Salem, drive 50 miles east on State Highway 22 to a junction immediately after a bridge over an arm of Detroit Reservoir and just before you enter the small town of Detroit. Turn left (northeast) on paved Forest Road 46, following signs to Breitenbush, go 11.9 miles, and then turn right on gravel Forest Road 4685. Stay on the main road for 7.5 miles to a fork. Go straight, still on Road 4685, and proceed 1.1 miles to the road-end parking area and trailhead.

Hiking It

From its start in a recovering clear-cut, the initially rocky trail ascends rapidly past young noble firs, mountain hemlocks, and lodgepole and western white pines. In late June of favorable years, this mostly open area is carpeted with an impressive display of thousands of tall beargrass blossoms. After 0.3 mile the steep uphill ends when you leave the clear-cut, enter the Mount Jefferson Wilderness, and begin to climb at a much gentler grade. Huckleberries line the path providing a tasty treat in late summer.

As it traverses near the top of a minor ridge the trail twice emerges from the forest to nice viewpoints where you can look down to the sparkling Fire-camp Lakes and see southeast to the towering summit of glacier-clad Mt. Jefferson.

The trail's last 0.3 mile is a gradual downhill across rocky, mostly open slopes. At 1.2 miles you reach a spacious campsite on the north shore of Crown Lake, the largest in the Firecamp Lakes chain. This shallow but lovely lake is surrounded by forest and has a view of the top third of Mt. Jefferson. The trail continues to the left, working around the north and east sides of the lake to another good campsite on the east shore.

From Crown Lake a sometimes sketchy boot path continues southeast to Claggett and Sheep lakes, the two smaller and slightly higher lakes in the chain. Since the trail beyond Crown Lake is not maintained and is often faint, you should be prepared to navigate with map and compass to reach these lakes.

All of the Firecamp Lakes are attractive and support either rainbow or brook trout. Unfortunately, Crown Lake is so shallow it is prone to freezing nearly to its bottom, thus killing almost all of the fish. As a result, this lake is no longer stocked. Claggett Lake is deeper and more reliable for both fishing and swimming. Sheep Lake is also fairly shallow and a bit brushy, but it has some really big trout.

58 Jefferson Park

RATINGS	Scenery **10** Difficulty **5 to 7** Solitude **2**
ROUND-TRIP DISTANCE	11.8 miles via Whitewater Trail; 13 miles via PCT from the north
ELEVATION GAIN	1900 feet via Whitewater Trail; 2700 feet via PCT
OPTIONAL MAPS	*Green Trails*: Breitenbush, Mount Jefferson
USUALLY OPEN	Mid-July to October
BEST TIMES	Late July to mid-August
AGENCY	Detroit Ranger District (Willamette National Forest) and Clackamas River Ranger District (Mount Hood National Forest)
PERMIT	Required. Free at the trailhead. Northwest Forest Pass required.

Highlights

Many seasoned backpackers contend that Jefferson Park is Oregon's most outstanding backcountry location. Certainly this alpine wonderland, with its wildflowers, tree islands, small lakes, and drop-dead-gorgeous views of nearby Mt. Jefferson, has few, if any, equals. But if you visit here, do not expect to be alone, because lots of other folks have heard about Jefferson Park as well. To protect this fragile area, the Forest Service requires that you camp only at sites that are designated by wooden posts. If possible, you should time your visit for midweek. The most popular access route is from the west along the Whitewater Trail, but if you don't mind a bumpy drive, it is much more scenic to come in via the Pacific Crest Trail (PCT) from the north. The view along the way from the top of

Jefferson Park

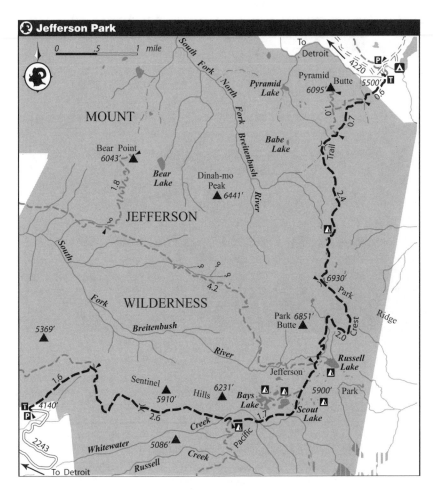

Park Ridge may be the finest viewpoint in the state of Oregon.

Getting There

From Salem, drive 50 miles east on State Highway 22 to a junction immediately after a bridge over an arm of Detroit Reservoir and just before you enter the small town of Detroit.

To reach the PCT Trailhead, turn left (northeast) onto paved Forest Road 46, following signs to Breitenbush, and drive 16.9 miles to a ridgetop junction with Road 4220. Turn right (east)

and drive 1 mile to a gate, where the gravel road changes to dirt. From here, the road is bumpy and rough, but it remains passable if you drive slowly. The signed trailhead is on the right, 5.5 miles from the gate.

If you are taking the Whitewater Trail from the west, continue on Highway 22 from Detroit another 10.4 miles, and then fork left onto wide, gravel Whitewater Road (Forest Road 2243). Follow this road for 7.4 miles to the large parking lot at a road-end clear-cut.

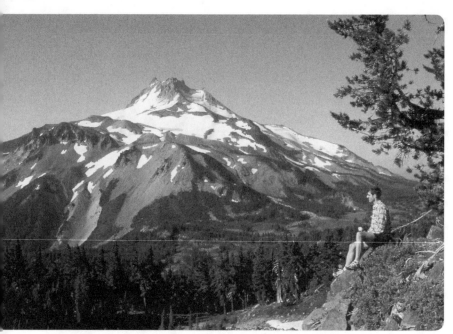

Mount Jefferson from Park Ridge east of the PCT, Mount Jeffeson Wilderness

Hiking It

Northern (PCT) Option: The PCT winds its way south through a delightful landscape of meadows filled with heather, huckleberries, and open forests dominated by mountain hemlocks. To the west you can see prominent Pyramid Butte. At 0.6 mile, keep left at an unsigned fork and continue through forest that gradually opens up to wildflower meadows. After passing through an indistinct pass, the trail wanders south, slowly gaining elevation as it passes through a land that is increasingly dominated by rocks and snow patches. You pass a campsite beside a small pond at 2.7 miles, and then ascend a large, semipermanent snowfield to the top of Park Ridge.

On a clear day, the view from here surpasses anything I could possibly describe. In the foreground, almost 900

feet below you, is the flat expanse of lake-dotted Jefferson Park, while rising impressively above the park is towering Mt. Jefferson, with its mantle of glaciers. You have to see this place to really appreciate it.

Once you have had your fill of this view, walk 2 miles down the well-graded trail in two long switchbacks to Russell Lake at the north end of Jefferson Park. Designated campsites are scattered around this and all the other lakes in the park, but the most scenic ones are those at Russell and Scout lakes. If you prefer a bit of solitude, try exploring the trailless eastern part of the park. This area has lesser views of the mountain, but plenty of wildflowers and some lovely little ponds.

Western (Whitewater Trail) Option: The trail soon climbs out of the rather unattractive old clear-cut at the trailhead and makes a steady, moderately graded climb in Douglas-fir forest for 1.6 miles to a ridgetop junction. Go right on the main trail and continue uphill, although now less steeply, winding your way south and east through a high-elevation forest of true firs and mountain hemlocks. After passing through a minor saddle, the trail levels out and crosses a partly open hillside on the south side of the ridge containing the Sentinel Hills. The openings along this scenic section provide outstanding views of Mt. Jefferson, with the shimmering masses of Russell and Jefferson Park glaciers on its flanks.

At 4.1 miles you cross Whitewater Creek in the middle of a small, wildflower-covered meadow, and soon reach a junction with the PCT. There is a nice campsite near this junction. You turn left (northbound) on the PCT and gradually climb through forest and small meadows, crossing Whitewater Creek a second time before leveling out as you enter the southwest part of Jefferson Park. The trail soon passes unsigned side trails that go left to Scout Lake and explore all the other wonders of this alpine paradise.

59 Pamelia and Shale Lakes Loop

RATINGS	Scenery **8** Difficulty **3 to 7** Solitude **3**
ROUND-TRIP DISTANCE	4.4 miles to Pamelia Lake; 17.7 miles for Shale Lake loop
ELEVATION GAIN	800 feet to Pamelia Lake; 3000 feet for Shale Lake Loop
OPTIONAL MAP	*Green Trails*: Mount Jefferson
USUALLY OPEN	Late May to late October to Pamelia Lake; mid-July to October for Shale Lake loop
BEST TIMES	Late July to mid-August
AGENCY	Detroit Ranger District (Willamette National Forest)
PERMIT	Required. Limited and advanced reservations are advised. Northwest Forest Pass required.
RESERVATION INFORMATION	The Forest Service has imposed a limited-entry permit system to protect the overused Pamelia Lake basin. Between the Friday of Memorial Day weekend and October 31, all hikers entering this area must obtain a free permit. These are available from the Detroit Ranger Station, either by phone or in person, within 30 days of your planned visit. Weekends in July and August are the most popular, so try to reserve as early as possible. For further information, go to www.fs.fed.us/r6/willamette/general/passespermits/recpasses/wilderness.html.

to Pamelia Lake

Highlights

Although there is a better view of Mt. Jefferson over Jefferson Park (Trip 58), the view from Shale Lake comes in a solid second place. That alone would make a visit here worthwhile, but this hike offers many other benefits. First, there is deservedly popular Pamelia Lake, a large, lower-elevation gem that is accessible from May to November.

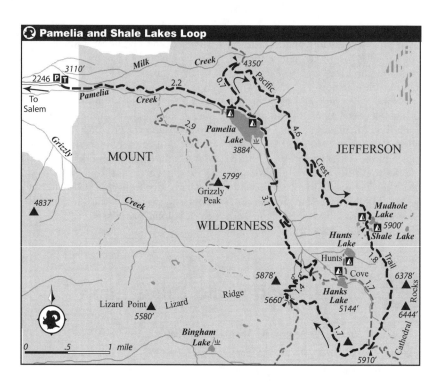

Pamelia and Shale Lakes Loop

Next, there are the stupendous views of Mt. Jefferson from the trail on the ridge south of Hunts Cove, as well as fine views of both the Cathedral Rocks and jagged Goat Peak. Finally, there are plenty of wildflower-covered meadows and lovely forests along the route. Overall, this is one of the better mountain loop hikes in our area.

Getting There

From Salem, drive 60 miles east on State Highway 22 to a junction between Mileposts 62 and 63. Turn left (east) on single-lane, paved Pamelia Creek Road (Forest Road 2246) and drive 2.9 miles to a junction. Go straight and proceed 0.9 mile on gravel to the road-end trailhead.

Hiking It

The wide trail's first 2.2 miles are a pleasant walk through a shady, old-growth forest of western red cedars, western hemlocks, and Douglas firs. Adding to the ambiance is cascading Pamelia Creek, which is always nearby to soothe hikers with its "river music." This gentle hike ends at a four-way junction immediately before you reach the northwest tip of Pamelia Lake. There are fine camps along the north shore of this 45-acre lake, although the water level often drops 10 to 20 feet by late summer, making the lake less attractive.

If you are doing the loop, turn left at the junction and climb away from the lake for 0.1 mile to a second junction. Go left again and ascend in a long curve through forest for 0.6 mile to a junction with the Pacific Crest Trail (PCT). Turn right (southbound) and make a long, gradual, switchbacking ascent through forest and past a couple of open areas where you can look down to Pamelia Lake. Eventually, you enter more interesting high-elevation terrain with open forests and small wildflower-covered meadows. At 7.5 miles you reach shallow Mudhole Lake and, just beyond, deeper but smaller Shale Lake. There are superb views to the north across these lakes to pointed Mt. Jefferson. You can also look east to ruggedly scenic Goat Peak. Camps are plentiful and very popular, especially with thru-hikers on the PCT. The best sites are along the west side of Mudhole Lake and on a low rise between the two lakes.

From Shale Lake the southbound PCT passes a couple of small ponds, visits a fine clifftop viewpoint over Hunts Cove, and then cuts across the west side of the rugged Cathedral Rocks. At 9.3 miles you come to a junction at a wide saddle, with a terrific view looking north to Mt. Jefferson over an area of red cinders. An old and now unmaintained trail goes north down the gully containing the red cinders, on its way to Hanks Lake. This is a somewhat shorter but less scenic alternative to the recommended loop.

The recommended route turns right (west) at the junction and loops around the south side of a little butte before coming out on the northeast side of a ridge and traversing an open slope with stupendous views to the north of Mt. Jefferson. After an all-too-short 0.5 mile, the trail crosses back over the ridge and drops to a junction in a saddle. You turn right and descend a series

of relatively short switchbacks for 1.4 miles to a junction with the spur trail into Hunts Cove. If you have the time, this side trail is worth taking to visit popular Hanks and Hunts lakes, both of which feature fine campsites but no views of Mt. Jefferson.

To complete the loop, take the trail that goes left (north) from the junction with the Hunts Cove Trail and drop steadily in long traverses and switchbacks to a crossing of Hunts Creek. You then gradually descend to Pamelia Lake, passing fine camps along its north shore, back to the junction at the northwest corner of that large lake. Go straight and return the 2.2 miles to your car.

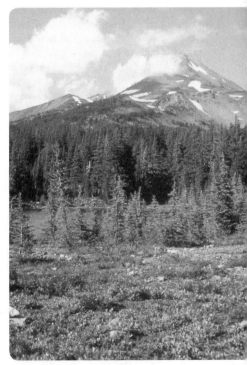

Mount Jefferson over Mudhole Lake

60 Carl Lake Loop

RATINGS	Scenery **7** Difficulty **4 to 6** Solitude **5**
ROUND-TRIP DISTANCE	9.8 miles to Carl Lake; 15.6 miles for the loop (plus explorations)
ELEVATION GAIN	1000 feet to Carl Lake; 1900 feet for the loop
OPTIONAL MAPS	*Green Trails: Mount Jefferson, Whitewater River*
USUALLY OPEN	Mid-July to October
BEST TIMES	Late July to mid-August
AGENCY	Sisters Ranger District (Deschutes National Forest)
PERMIT	Required. Free at the trailhead.

Highlights

A deep, sparkling jewel set beneath a particularly rugged and scenic stretch of the Cascade Mountains, Carl Lake is a fun destination for an overnight trip in the central Mount Jefferson Wilderness. Adventurous hikers can make this into a semiloop trip by seeking out an unofficial path up to the Pacific Crest Trail (PCT), with the option to do a bit of off-trail exploring. Although never very steep or difficult, the trail into Carl Lake travels through a large burn area that can be hot on summer afternoons.

Getting There

From Santiam Pass, 89 miles east of Salem, go east 7.6 miles on U.S. Highway 20 to the signed junction with paved Jack Lake Road (Forest Road 12). Turn left (north), following signs to Mt. Jefferson Wilderness trailheads, drive 4.4 miles, and then go left on single-lane paved Road 1230. Proceed 1.8 miles, and then go right at a junction, staying on Road 1230, which now turns to gravel. Remain on Road 1230 through several minor intersections for 4.9 miles, and then fork left and proceed a

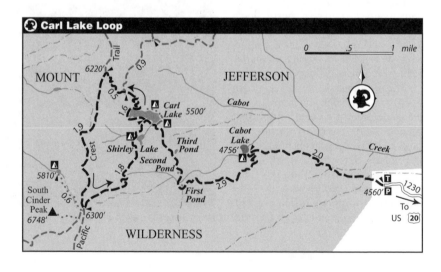

final 2 miles to the signed Cabot Lake Trailhead.

Hiking It

Starting in a recent burn area, the often dusty trail wanders intermittently uphill past blackened snags and a few living conifers. Without the usual forest cover, the vegetation here consists of shrubs such as deer brush, huckleberries, and red-flowering currant, as well as sun-loving wildflowers like pearly everlasting, beardtongue, and (not surprisingly) fireweed.

At 1.5 miles you leave the burn zone and enter a beautiful, shady forest that features a mix of mountain hemlocks, western white pines, lodgepole pines, Engelmann spruces, and a few ponderosa pines. At 2 miles an obvious but unsigned spur trail goes downhill to the right to forest- and marsh-rimmed Cabot Lake, a pleasant but viewless pool with decent campsites.

After the Cabot Lake turnoff, the main trail begins a sustained ascent, climbing a mostly forested hillside in 12 well-graded switchbacks. Once the switchbacks end, you continue uphill for another 0.5 mile, and then meander past a series of small lakelets with the rather unimaginative names of First, Second, and Third ponds. Finally, at 4.8 miles you reach the southeast end of Carl Lake. This deep, oval-shaped lake has a rocky shoreline and numerous possible campsites. The most popular sites are near the trail on the south side of the lake, but the most scenic sites are on the east and north shores, where you can look across the water to the crags along the Cascade divide. The east shore sites are easy to reach along an unsigned but obvious spur trail, but those along the north shore require a bit of relatively easy scrambling.

The main trail goes through the forest on the south shore of Carl Lake to a junction with the trail to Shirley Lake. This is the return route of the recommended loop. Since the loop is easier to navigate if you travel counterclockwise, go straight on the main trail as it loops around the west side of Carl Lake, and then ascends 20 well-graded switchbacks to a tiny, shallow pond. Immediately past this pond is an unsigned fork. The main trail goes straight, but you turn left and follow a winding and unofficial trail as it steeply ascends for 0.5 mile to the top of the divide and an unsigned junction with the Pacific Crest Trail. Turn left (south) on this very scenic trail as it goes up and down along the ridge, passing excellent viewpoints of such landmarks as South Cinder Peak to the south and pointed Mt. Jefferson to the north. In one or two places you can also look east down to sparkling Carl Lake. After 1.9 miles you come to a saddle and a four-way junction.

The trail back to Carl Lake goes left, but if you have some extra time and energy, consider doing some relatively easy cross-country exploring. One excellent option is the scramble up South Cinder Peak, the prominent, reddish cinder cone that rises to the southwest. The route to the view-packed summit is open and easy to negotiate. Another possible destination is a small but scenic unnamed lake at the northern base of South Cinder Peak. To reach it, go northwest from the pass down a steep, forested hillside into a prominent drainage. Once on the bottom, head downstream on a sketchy and intermittent bootpath that travels gradually downhill through forests and flower-covered meadows for 0.5 mile to the meadow-rimmed little lake. There is a good campsite at the lake's west end,

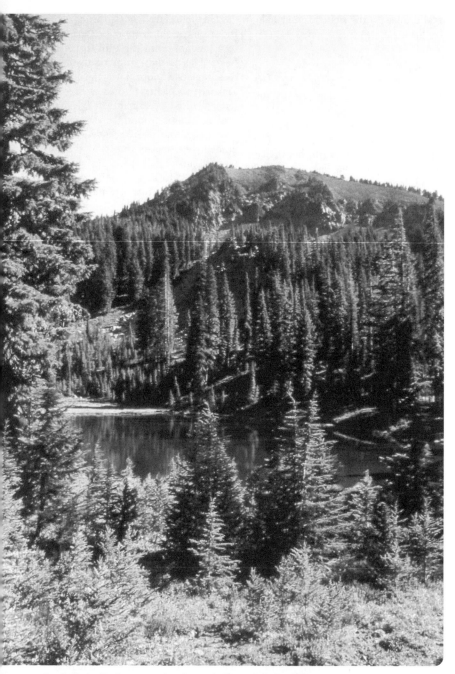

South Cinder Peak over pond to the north, Mount Jefferson Wilderness which provides a less crowded alternative to spending the night at popular Carl Lake.

Once you've had your fill of exploring, head northeast from the four-way junction at the pass and descend a good trail that crosses a mostly open hillside with good views of Mt. Jefferson and the nearby crags of the Cascade divide. After 1.4 miles you pass irregularly shaped Shirley Lake, which has decent campsites, and return to Carl Lake. Turn right and retrace your steps back to the trailhead.

61   Duffy and Santiam Lakes

RATINGS	Scenery **8** Difficulty **3 to 4** Solitude **5**
ROUND-TRIP DISTANCE	7 miles to Duffy Lake; 9.6 miles to Santiam Lake
ELEVATION GAIN	800 feet to Duffy Lake; 1200 feet to Santiam Lake
OPTIONAL MAP	*U.S. Forest Service: Mount Jefferson Wilderness*
USUALLY OPEN	Mid-June to October
BEST TIMES	July (but be prepared for mosquitoes)
AGENCY	Detroit Ranger District (Willamette National Forest)
PERMIT	Required. Free at the trailhead. Northwest Forest Pass required.

Highlights

The forested terrain of the southern Mount Jefferson Wilderness is dominated by two outstanding features, the rugged crags of Three Fingered Jack and the tranquil beauty of dozens of mountain lakes. Both features are included in this relatively easy hike that visits two of the most attractive and popular lakes in this area. Forest-rimmed Duffy Lake has no good view of Three Fingered Jack, but features fine camps and a nice view of pointed Duffy Butte. Santiam Lake, on the other hand, sits in

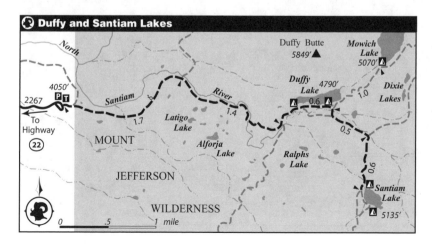

Duffy and Santiam Lakes

a meadow basin and has a great view of Three Fingered Jack, in fact one of the best anywhere of this impressive mountain. Although huge fires swept through this area in 2003, most of the damage occurred north and east of the trails described here. Only a few places along this route display evidence of the fire, so the hiking remains scenic and the forests green.

Getting There

From Salem, drive east on State Highway 22 to Milepost 76, then turn left (east) on one-lane paved Big Meadows Road (Forest Road 2267). Stay on the main road for 3.1 miles to the trailhead.

Hiking It

The trail goes east at a gentle grade through forest, soon meeting an equestrian trail that starts at a different trailhead. Go straight and continue with your gradual uphill, passing a spring at 1.1 miles and coming to a junction with the Turpentine Trail at 1.7 miles. Go straight and soon level off as you proceed through a lovely mix of forest and meadows along the sluggish headwaters of the North Santiam River. After making an easy but unbridged crossing of the tiny "river," you proceed through more meadows to a junction at 3.1 miles.

Go straight on the more heavily used trail and walk another 0.4 mile, mostly on the level, to a junction near the southwest corner of long, clear Duffy Lake. There is a good campsite not far to the left here, and more sites on the north and southeast shores. The ridge north of Duffy Lake, which is dominated by the pyramid-shaped summit of rocky Duffy Butte, is covered

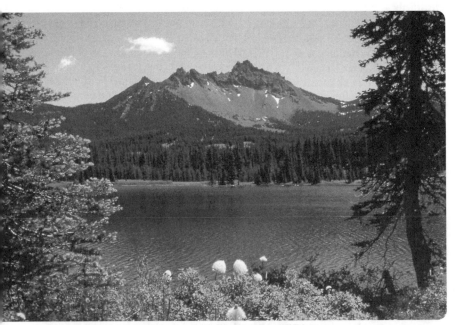

Three Fingered Jack over Santiam Lake, Mount Jeffeson Wilderness

with blackened snags from the huge 2003 B&B Complex Fire. Fortunately, although there is spotty fire damage nearer the trail, the south side of Duffy Lake generally escaped the flames.

After making a bridged crossing of Duffy Lake's often-dry outlet creek, you come to a junction. The trail going straight leads to Mowich Lake and the fire-ravaged Eight Lakes Basin. To reach Santiam Lake, turn right and soon come to a second junction. Turn left and gradually ascend to a junction in a lovely meadow that in July is covered with a beautiful display of pink shooting stars.

Turn right at the junction and climb on a badly eroded trail for 0.6 mile to spectacular, meadow-rimmed Santiam Lake. There are several excellent camps near this lake, all of which provide outstanding views across the water to jagged Three Fingered Jack. In July the scene is particularly beautiful, with lots of wildflowers in the foreground and plenty of snow still on the peak. Unfortunately, that is also mosquito time, and the nasty little vampires are both abundant and mean. By mid-August most of the bugs are gone, but so are the flowers. Take your pick.

62 Three Fingered Jack Loop

RATINGS	Scenery **9** Difficulty **8** Solitude **5**
ROUND-TRIP DISTANCE	20.5 miles
ELEVATION GAIN	3300 feet
OPTIONAL MAP	*U.S. Forest Service: Mount Jefferson Wilderness*
USUALLY OPEN	Mid-July to October
BEST TIMES	Late July
AGENCY	Detroit Ranger District (Willamette National Forest) and Sisters Ranger District (Deschutes National Forest)
PERMIT	Required. Free at the trailhead. Northwest Forest Pass required.

Highlights

A jagged sentinel for much of the central Oregon Cascades, Three Fingered Jack is all that remains of an extinct volcano that has eroded away, leaving only the hard central plug of lava. Scenic trails go almost all the way around the mountain, offering excellent views, visiting small lakes, and taking the hiker through some of the best wildflower fields in Oregon. Part of the recommended loop involves some easy cross-country travel, but that should not deter experienced hikers. Literalists beware, however, because despite the mountain's name, even after walking the entire loop and seeing the peak from every angle, it is hard to figure out from just where it supposedly has three "fingers." Actually the name's origin is unknown and may refer to an early trapper with somewhat fewer than the usual number of digits.

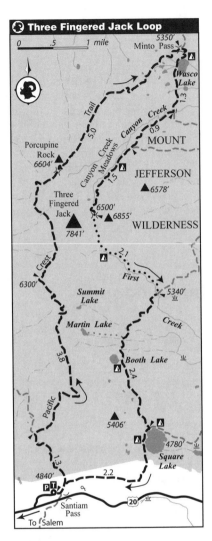

Three Fingered Jack Loop

0   .5   1 mile

5350'
Minto Pass

Wasco Lake

Canyon Creek Trail

Canyon Creek Meadows

Porcupine Rock 6604'

Three Fingered Jack 7841'

6500'
6855'

MOUNT JEFFERSON
6578'

WILDERNESS

Pacific Crest

6300'

Summit Lake

First

5340'

Martin Lake

Creek

Booth Lake

5406'

4780'
Square Lake

4840'

2.2

Santiam Pass

20

To Salem

Getting There

From Salem, drive 83 miles east on State Highway 22 to where it merges with U.S. Highway 20, and then continue east another 6 miles to a signed junction with the spur road to the Pacific Crest Trailhead just west of Santiam Pass. Turn left and proceed 0.2 mile to the large trailhead parking lot.

Hiking It

From the parking lot you follow a short spur trail that goes east to a junction with the Pacific Crest Trail (PCT) and turn left (north). This wide trail winds gradually uphill through what used to be an open forest of lodgepole pines and true firs with an abundance of beargrass covering the forest floor. After the huge B&B Complex Fire swept through this area in 2003, however, many of the trees became blackened snags. This makes for hot, shadeless hiking, but provides for better views and more life-giving sunshine for wildflowers. You will be going in and out of the fire zone for most of this trip.

After 0.2 mile you pass a poorly signed junction with the trail going right (east) to Square Lake, which will be your return trail if you do the recommended loop. Keep straight on the PCT and continue uphill, mostly through burned areas and past a couple of stagnant lily-pad-covered ponds to a junction at 1.3 miles. Go right, still on the PCT, and keep going steadily but not steeply uphill.

At about 3.8 miles, just as you leave the burn zone, you pass the first nice viewpoint of Three Fingered Jack, which looks like a single tall spire from this angle. Another first-rate viewpoint comes at 4.6 miles when you pass a rocky outcropping on the left (southwest) side of the trail. The view to the south from here of Mt. Washington, the Three Sisters, and for miles beyond is breathtaking. The best view of all, however, comes at 5.1 miles when you round a corner and are suddenly faced with an up-close view of the huge west face of Three Fingered Jack. Snow streaks the slopes of the mountain into August, making this view even more photogenic.

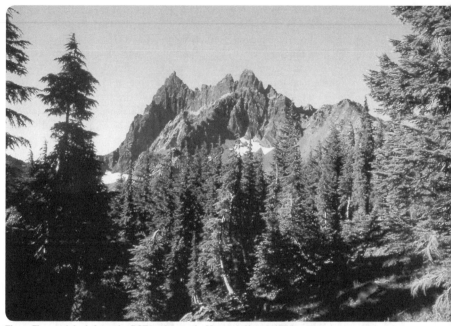

Three Fingered Jack from the PCT to the north, Mount Jefferson Wilderness

The PCT now contours across the west side of Three Fingered Jack, mostly across rocky slopes. There are nice views to the west here of the forests and burned areas around Santiam Lake. At 6.9 miles you go through a little pass next to Porcupine Rock, and then make a few downhill switchbacks across an open slope. The views here looking south to nearby Three Fingered Jack are outstanding, especially highlighting the dark bands of red and black rock that make up the jagged mountain. From here the trail slowly descends, mostly in forest and areas that show spotty effects of the fires. Finally, you circle around a series of shallow ponds before coming to Minto Pass and a junction at 10.1 miles. Turn right, leaving the PCT, and descend a fairly steep trail to clear Wasco Lake. The Forest Service requires that

overnight visitors use designated campsites located along this lake's north and east sides.

The trail goes south along the west shore of Wasco Lake, and then travels through forest to a junction immediately after you cross Canyon Creek. There is a small but attractive waterfall just below this crossing. Turn right at this junction and make your way gradually upstream, passing old beaver ponds along the way, to a junction near the lower end of Canyon Creek Meadows. Turn right and wind your way gradually through these gorgeous meadows that in late July feature incredible displays of lupine, monkeyflower, paintbrush, and other wildflowers. In the upper parts of the meadows there are some terrific views of Three Fingered Jack. After leaving the meadows the trail climbs through a rocky area and then steeply ascends along the top of an old moraine above a tiny lake to a wind-swept pass directly beneath the sheer cliffs of Three Fingered Jack.

The trail ends at the pass. To complete the recommended loop, carefully pick your way down the steep, rocky slope on the south side of the pass to a rather barren, pumice-covered meadow at the head of trickling First Creek. There are some excellent and extremely scenic camps in the trees at the edge of this meadow. From here you continue going cross-country, following the creek downstream mostly through large burn areas. Be prepared to hike over or around some deadfall in this area. About 0.5 mile below the first meadow, look for a shallow pond a little northeast of the creek. This pond provides terrific early-morning reflections of Three Fingered Jack. About 0.6 mile below the pond you intersect a maintained trail.

Turn right on the trail and go mostly downhill through forest and burn areas, crossing several seasonal creeks along the way to pleasant Booth Lake at 17 miles. This lake has nice campsites and is good for swimming. To close the loop, continue south another 1.3 miles to a junction at large and popular Square Lake (more camps). Turn right and close out the loop with a 2-mile stroll through forest and burn areas back to the junction with the PCT just 0.2 mile from the trailhead. Turn left and return to your car.

63 Washington Ponds and George Lake

RATINGS	Scenery **7** Difficulty **5 to 7** Solitude **7**
ROUND-TRIP DISTANCE	12 miles to Washington Ponds; 17.5 miles to George Lake
ELEVATION GAIN	1150 feet to Washington Ponds; 1600 feet to George Lake
OPTIONAL MAP	*U.S. Forest Service: Mount Washington Wilderness*
USUALLY OPEN	Mid-June to October
BEST TIMES	Late June and July
AGENCY	McKenzie River Ranger District (Willamette National Forest) and Sisters Ranger District (Deschutes National Forest)
PERMIT	Required. Free at the trailhead.

Highlights

In its long course from Mexico to Canada, the Pacific Crest Trail (PCT) takes hikers high on the slopes of many of the northwest's famous volcanic peaks, providing fine views and excellent mountain scenery. One of the lesser known of those peaks is pointed Mt. Washington, which rises above a land of rolling forests and vast lava flows in the central Oregon Cascades. But "lesser known" is not the same as less beautiful, as this section of that famous trail amply demonstrates. The views and scenery here are perhaps not as spec-

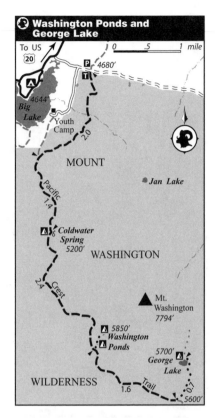

Washington Ponds and George Lake

To US 20

P 4680'

Big Lake 4644'

Youth Camp

2.0

MOUNT

● Jan Lake

Pacific 1.4

Coldwater Spring 5200'

WASHINGTON

Crest 2.4

▲ Mt. Washington 7794'

5850'
Washington Ponds

5700'
George Lake

WILDERNESS

Trail 1.6

0.7

5600'

the junction with the Big Lake Road at Milepost 80 just before you reach Santiam Pass. Turn right (south), drive 1 mile, and then veer left at the junction with the road into Hoodoo Ski Area. Drive 2.2 miles and then go left on a rough gravel road, following signs to Pacific Crest Youth Camp. After 0.4 mile you go straight where the main road turns right and proceed 0.2 mile on a rough dirt road to the trailhead on the right.

Hiking It

The well-graded Pacific Crest Trail (PCT) goes south through a rather monotonous and viewless forest of lodgepole pines and mountain hemlocks. The route is generally either level or very gradually uphill for the first 2 miles until you come to an unsigned but obvious junction with a wide and dusty trail that goes sharply right toward a youth camp. Continue south on the PCT, which remains in forest, but now steadily climbs, gaining a little over 400 feet in 1.4 miles to the small meadow holding Coldwater Spring. There is a camp just beyond the spring on the right (west) side of the trail and a partial view over the meadow of the summit spire of Mt. Washington. Unfortunately, the often muddy spring is rather unattractive and overused by climbers, backpackers, and horse parties. By late summer the spring may dry up.

For better scenery and better camping options, continue on the PCT as it gains elevation, and at 5 miles crosses the rocky south side of an open ridge. Here you are greeted with the first really good views of the trip. Especially impressive are the vistas to the south over the huge McKenzie lava flows to Belknap Crater, the Three Sisters, and

tacular as those around Mt. Jefferson or Mt. Hood, but they are still mighty impressive and well worth seeing. The biggest drawback to backpacking this section of the PCT is a lack of water. The only reliable water sources are the two small Washington Ponds and larger and more attractive George Lake. Both of these locations are off the main trail, which makes them harder to find, but provides greater solitude.

Getting There

From Salem, drive 83 miles east on State Highway 22 to where it merges with U.S. Highway 20 and continue east on that route another 6 miles to distant Diamond Peak. The hiking is now delightful, as the trail soon leaves the rocky slope and rounds a little basin that features an open forest of mountain hemlocks and subalpine firs and a cinder-covered meadow with outstanding views up to the jagged spire of nearby Mt. Washington. About 0.2 mile beyond the end of the meadow is a normally dry gully. Look carefully here for an unsigned and hard-to-locate route that goes left (north-northeast) about 250 yards to shallow Lower Washington Pond. This pond has a decent view of the top third of Mt. Washington and a pleasant camp on some flat ground above its west shore. Locating more attractive Upper Washington Pond requires a bit of exploring, as the trail to it is sketchy and often disappears. To find it, go north then northeast up a steep little slope for about 0.2 mile and look for the small basin holding the pond. There is a nice campsite above the water's northwest shore. Both of the Washington Ponds are more attractive in early summer when the water is high and fresh from new snowmelt.

The hike's best camps and water, however, are at George Lake. To find this lake, continue south on the PCT, going gradually downhill through forest for 1.6 miles, and then leave the trail about 0.4 mile before you round the end of a large lava flow. The route is cross-country, but you may see a faint tread in places or pick out a few orange flags to guide you along the way. The best way to find the lake is to go very gradually uphill, heading north-northeast over a forested ridge until you see the shimmering lake in the basin to the north. Drop down to its welcome waters and set up camp above the northeast shore. The lake

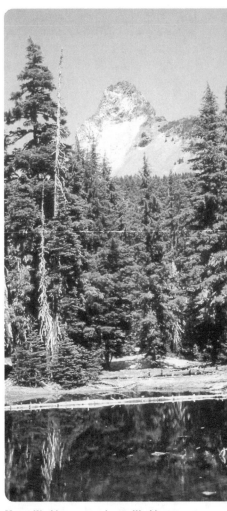

Mount Washington over Lower Washington Pond

has excellent and reliable water and is fine for swimming. It also features a superb view of the towering summit spire of Mt. Washington. For an even better view, scramble to the top of a ridge about 0.4 mile north of George Lake where you gain a terrific perspective of the impressive east face of Mt. Washington.

64 Cache Creek

RATINGS	Scenery **7** Difficulty **5** Solitude **9**
ROUND-TRIP DISTANCE	5.5 miles
ELEVATION GAIN	900 feet
OPTIONAL MAP	*USGS: Mount Washington*
USUALLY OPEN	Late June to October
BEST TIMES	July
AGENCY	Sisters Ranger District (Deschutes National Forest)
PERMIT	Required. Free at the trailhead.

Highlights

The steep eastern face of Mt. Washington is familiar to countless thousands of drivers who have admired this pointed mountain from the popular viewpoint on U.S. Highway 20 above Suttle Lake. Almost none of those camera-toting tourists, however, have attempted to get a closer look at this impressive peak. This is understandable, since no official trail reaches the scenic, sloping meadows beneath the mountain's eastern cliffs. But adventuresome hikers who are willing to seek out a sketchy climber's trail can access this area and be rewarded with a night in one of the most impressive locations in central Oregon. Make this trip early in the summer, however, since Cache Creek (the only source of water) may dry up by late summer.

Getting There

From Santiam Pass, 89 miles east of Salem, drive 8.1 miles east on U.S. Highway 20, and then turn right (south) on gravel Forest Road 2067. Drive 0.2 mile to a fork, go left, and then stay on Road 2067 for 5.3 miles to a junction. Go straight on Road 500, following signs to Hortense Lake, and proceed 3.2 miles to the signed trailhead on the left. The last 0.2 mile of this road is rather rough.

Hiking It

After obtaining a free permit at the trailhead, hike south on a little-used trail through an open forest of mountain hemlocks, western white pines, and true firs. Unfortunately, the trail soon leaves this shady forest and enters a burn area, where blackened snags despoil the scenery and deadfall often blocks the trail. Expect to make short detours around downed logs or scramble over the deadfall. At 1.6 miles you reenter forest and come to a log crossing of seasonal Cache Creek.

The official trail goes straight, but to find the unmaintained use path up Cache Creek, backtrack about 25 yards and pick up an unsigned trail that goes upstream. This trail has a few old cut logs to help keep you on course, but it is still faint and has some deadfall. Fortunately the winding path is always just a short distance from Cache Creek, making the tread easy to relocate if lost. The trail is steep at times, but is always enjoyable as it follows the cascading little creek.

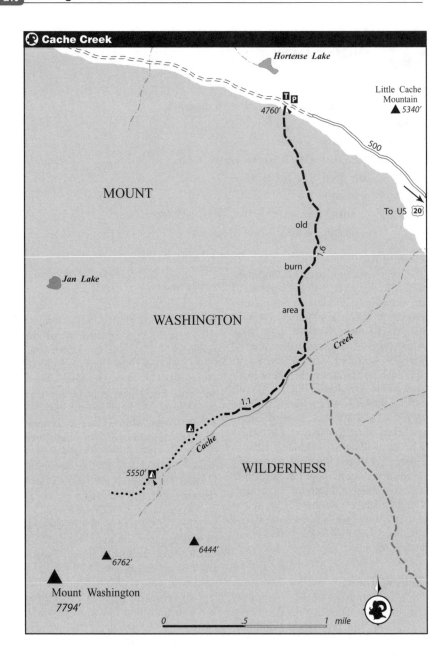

Cache Creek

Hortense Lake

Little Cache
Mountain
▲ 5340'

4760'

500

MOUNT

To US 20

old

1.6

burn

Jan Lake

WASHINGTON

area

Creek

1.1

Cache

5550'

WILDERNESS

6444'

6762'

Mount Washington
7794'

0   .5   1 mile

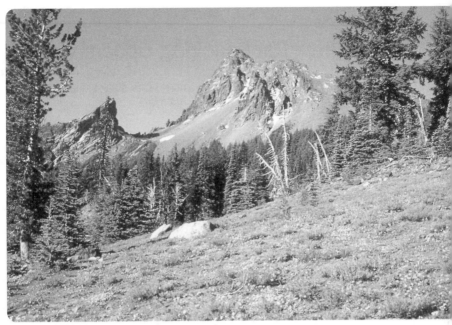

Mount Washington from meadows to the east, Mount Washington Wilderness

After a little over 0.7 mile, the country opens up, the trail peters out, and you pass a couple of excellent possible campsites under the shade of some large mountain hemlock trees. More possible campsites are found about 0.4 mile upstream.

To find the best photo spots, keep going west-southwest (uphill) and wander around the trailless terrain north of the creek, passing through several sloping, pumice-covered meadows that provide views of the massive east face of Mt. Washington. The rewards for this effort are considerable, with numerous great spots to sit, eat lunch, and enjoy the scenery. Just southeast of the mountain's main summit is a sharp, colorfully striated, unnamed pinnacle that adds to the scenery. Solitude is another bonus as typically the only other users of this unofficial trail are the few climbers who tackle the difficult east face of Mount Washington.

APPENDIX A
More Short Backpacking Options

Southeastern Olympic Mountains

MILDRED LAKES
Round trip: 11 miles / 3000 feet

Fairly popular but very steep and rough, this boot-beaten path leads to a series of scenic subalpine lakes with fine views of rugged Sawtooth Ridge. The trail is poorly maintained and not suitable for children. Access is from the end of Forest Road 25 along the Hamma Hamma River (see Trip 2).

EAST FORK LENA CREEK
Round trip from the Lena Lake Trailhead: 13 miles / 2400 feet

An old climber's route (now a maintained trail) branches off from the north end of Lena Lake (see Trip 3) and ascends a deep valley to scenic camps beneath The Brothers. There are several creek crossings along the way.

FLAPJACK LAKES
Round trip: 15.6 miles / 3100 feet

A rather steep trail leads to two very popular lakes in the high country beneath rugged Sawtooth Ridge and Mt. Lincoln, with access to the lovely high country around Gladys Divide. The lakes are pretty, but not enough to explain their extreme popularity. Start from Staircase Ranger Station at the north end of Lake Cushman, which is accessed by a road that leaves U.S. Highway 101 at the town of Hoodsport. A limited access permit is required from Olympic National Park. Reservations are strongly advised.

NORTH FORK SKOKOMISH RIVER TRAIL
Round trip to the campsite at Nine Stream: 19.2 miles / 1300 feet (with shorter and longer options)

This gentle valley walk follows a well-maintained trail through beautiful old-growth forests. The route is fairly crowded and has no views, but is pleasant and is open for most of the year. The trail also provides access for longer trips to the beautiful alpine meadow at Home Sweet Home and beyond. Start from Staircase Ranger Station at the north end of Lake Cushman, which is accessed by a road that leaves U.S. Highway 101 at the town of Hoodsport. An Olympic National Park permit is required.

SOUTH FORK SKOKOMISH RIVER TRAIL
Round trip to Sundown Lake: 14.2 miles / 3200 feet (with many shorter options along the river)

A good trail through magnificent old-growth forest along a pretty stream and past pleasant, kid-friendly camps eventually turns into a rough, steep boot path into the high country. From Shelton, drive 7 miles north on U.S. Highway 101, and then turn left (west) on South Fork Skokomish Road, which eventually becomes gravel Forest Road 23. After 18 miles veer right on Road 2361 and follow this for 5.5 miles to its end. An Olympic National Park permit is required if you go as far as the camp at tiny Sundown Lake.

Southern Mount Rainier and the Goat Rocks

BERTHA MAY AND GRANITE LAKES

Round trip to Granite Lake: 3.3 miles / 750 feet

The attractions here are two very scenic lakes with fine camps and views of the impressive cliffs on the north side of Sawtooth Ridge. The trail also provides access to a longer trip into Cora Lake. Be prepared to encounter motorcycles, as this entire area is overrun with them. Drive as to Trip 4, but turn south off Highway 706 about 10.1 miles east of its junction with Highway 7 onto paved Forest Road 52. After 4.8 miles turn right (south) on gravel Road 84, go 1.6 miles, and then turn right on Forest Road 8410 for 3.9 miles to the Tealy Creek Trailhead.

KLAPATCHE PARK

Round trip: 18.5 miles / 3600 feet

A famous and breathtakingly beautiful site near tiny Aurora Lake in the alpine landscape on Mt. Rainier's west face. The trail is prone to washouts, and obtaining a permit for one of the two available campsites is tricky, but the scenery is worth it. The trail starts from the end of the washed-out and permanently closed West Side Road in the southwest part of Mount Rainier National Park. Hike along the closed road for 3 miles, then turn east on the South Puyallup River Trail past the Colonnades, an impressive basalt formation, to a junction with the Wonderland Trail. Turn left (north) and climb past pretty St. Andrews Lake to Klapatche Park. A Mount Rainier National Park permit is required and reservations are strongly recommended.

CAMP MUIR

Round trip: 10.5 miles / 4700 feet

A climber's camp perched at 10,100 feet on the south side of Mt. Rainier. The camp is exposed to the weather, crowded, and very smelly, but the views seem to extend forever. Considerable snow travel is required. Start at famous Paradise Lodge amid crowds of tourists and acres of flowers, before climbing high into the land of rocks and ice. A Mount Rainier National Park permit is required and reservations are helpful.

SNOW LAKE

Round trip: 2.2 miles / 250 feet

A small lake in a deep canyon below the pointed summit of Unicorn Peak. Although Snow Lake has no view of the park's namesake attraction, the gentle access trail passes wildflower meadows and Bench Lake, which features grand reflections of Mt. Rainier. A Mount Rainier National Park permit is required and reservations are recommended. The trail starts off the Stevens Canyon Road about 1.5 miles east of Reflection Lake.

JUG AND FRYINGPAN LAKES

Round trip to Fryingpan Lake: 9.8 miles / 1600 feet

Two fairly large and very pretty lakes in the southwestern William O. Douglas Wilderness that are very popular with equestrians. Jug Lake is rimmed with forest, while shallow Fryingpan Lake is in a large meadow. The trail provides access to the PCT and miles of excellent meadow walking with a possible loop that returns via Penoyer Creek. Expect clouds of mosquitoes in July. From Packwood, go 8.8 miles northeast on U.S. Highway 12, turn left on gravel Forest Road 4510, and drive 5 miles to its end at the Soda Springs Campground and Trailhead.

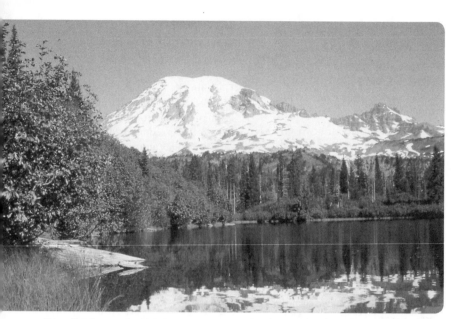

Mount Rainier over Bench Lake (on trail to Snow Lake), Mount Rainier National Park

BLUE LAKE

Round trip: 5.2 miles / 1800 feet

A steep, hiker-only path follows a creek up a narrow gorge past rock formations and viewpoints to a large and quite scenic lake in an unprotected roadless area south of Mt. Rainier. Unfortunately, the lake is also accessible via a separate motorcycle trail, so expect noisy machines at the destination. Take U.S. Highway 12 to a junction in Randle, turn right (south) for 1 mile, and then turn left on paved Road 23. Go 15.2 miles, and then turn left onto Road 171 and drive this steep gravel road 1.6 miles to the road-end trailhead.

McCALL BASIN VIA THE PACIFIC CREST TRAIL

Round trip to McCall Basin: 26.8 miles / 4300 feet

A very long but scenic high-elevation section of the Pacific Crest Trail south from White Pass leads past meadow-rimmed Shoe Lake to forested Tieton Pass and on to the excellent camps in McCall Basin. The best scenery is another 0.5 mile to the south along an unofficial trail into spectacular Glacier Basin. This hike is often done as part of a longer point-to-point trip along the PCT through the Goat Rocks Wilderness. Start from the PCT Trailhead just east of White Pass along U.S. Highway 12.

GLACIER LAKE

Round trip: 4 miles / 750 feet

A fairly large lake in the western Goat Rocks Wilderness that is backed by a long, forested ridge is the destination on this nicely shaded hike. The lake is uncrowded and offers good fishing, but the water level tends to recede significantly by midsummer making it less attractive. Drive 62 miles east on U.S. Highway 12 from Interstate 5, then turn right (south) on good gravel Forest Road 21. Go 5.1 miles, then turn left on Road 2110 and drive 0.5 mile on this steep and rocky road to the trailhead on the right.

NANNIE RIDGE LOOP

Round trip for loop: 14.2 miles / 2000 feet

A very scenic loop hike with excellent views and fine wildflower displays in the southern Goat Rocks Wilderness. The loop goes up rugged Nannie Ridge to a junction with the PCT and possible campsites at tiny Sheep Lake. A nice side trip goes north to spectacular Cispus Pass, but the main loop goes south, and then returns on a trail down Walupt Creek. Drive 62 miles east on U.S. Highway 12 from Interstate 5, then turn right (south) on good gravel Forest Road 21. Go 16.3 miles, then turn left (east) on one-lane paved Road 2160 and proceed 5 miles to the trailhead beside large and popular Walupt Lake.

Mount St. Helens Area

PLAINS OF ABRAHAM

Round trip as semiloop to camps at south end of Plains of Abraham: 11.8 miles / 1200 feet

A wildly scenic trail leads to a spectacular, desolate plain high on the eastern flank of Mt. St. Helens. Much of the route crosses the area devastated by the 1980 eruption, so there is almost no shade and no protection from the wind. Trail closures due to volcanic activity are common. The only legal camping is south of the plain near a seasonal creek just outside the devastated area. The trip is better when done as a semiloop

with a portion of the Loowit Trail over rugged Windy Pass. Drive as for Trip 13 to the junction of Roads 99 and 26, but go left (south) on Road 99 for 6.9 miles to the road-end parking lot on Windy Ridge.

BUTTE CAMP

Round trip to camp: 4.2 miles / 1000 feet

A lovely trail with great views of the south side of Mt. St. Helens climbs to a viewless camp below Butte Camp Dome. The trail provides access to great alpine scenery along the Loowit Trail and a less crowded (but longer) route to the top of the mountain than the popular Monitor Ridge route. A reserved permit is required to climb the mountain, but not to stay at the camp. From Interstate 5 at Woodland Exit 21 go 35 miles east on Highway 503 and 503 Spur to a junction about 6 miles past Cougar. Turn left on paved Road 83, go 3.1 miles, and then turn left on Road 81 and drive 1.4 miles to the trailhead at Redrock Pass. The final mile of the access road is subject to frequent washouts, so check on conditions before your visit.

SOUTH FORK TOUTLE RIVER

Round trip by most direct route: 10.4 miles / 2100 feet

Permanent road washouts have turned what used to be an easy dayhike on the west side of Mt. St. Helens into a longer backpacking trip with excellent views along the edge of the devastated area. Drive as to Butte Camp above, but continue past Redrock Pass another 2.3 miles to the junction with Road 8123, which is now closed. Walk up the road for 1.7 miles, then follow Blue Lake Trail to a campsite on a clear creek a little before you reach the stark canyon of silt-laden South Fork

Toutle River. The trip can also be done as a long, rugged loop trip from Butte Camp using a portion of the Loowit Trail to complete the loop.

JUNE LAKE

Round trip: 2.8 miles / 450 feet

A popular and easy hike on the forested south side of Mt. St. Helens to an interesting lake created by a mudflow. A scenic waterfall drops almost directly into the lake. From Interstate 5 at Woodland Exit 21 go 35 miles east on Highway 503 and 503 Spur to a junction about 6 miles past Cougar. Turn left on paved Road 83 and proceed 7 miles to the signed trailhead.

BADGER LAKE

Round trip to lake: 8.8 miles / 1000 feet

A tiny but pretty lake that sits in a meadowy basin along the Boundary Trail east of Mt. St. Helens. From the lake a side trail leads 0.9 mile to the outstanding views from the old lookout site atop Badger Peak. Sadly, the trails here are a playground for noisy, erosion-causing motorcycles, so be prepared to put up with machines. Drive as described in Trip 13 to the junction near Pine Creek Information Center. Go straight on Road 25 for 21.7 miles to the signed trailhead at Elk Pass.

Mount Adams and Indian Heaven

LOOKINGGLASS LAKE

Round Trip: 8.2 miles / 1450 feet

A pleasant ridge walk leads to a small lake in the southwestern Mount Adams Wilderness with nice camps and a partial view of the peak. Nearby Madcat Meadow features lots of flowers and better mountain views. Drive as

described in Trip 19 to the turnoff for Road 23 north of Trout Lake, but only stay on Road 23 for 8.8 miles before turning right on gravel Road 8031. Go 0.4 mile, turn left on rough Road 070 for 3.2 miles, and then turn right on Road 120 for 0.8 mile to the trailhead in an old clear-cut.

PLACID LAKE

Round trip: 1.6 miles / 100 feet

Short and nearly level trail to tranquil, forest-rimmed lake in the northwestern Indian Heaven Wilderness. The lake is ideal for fishing, swimming, and the quiet contemplation of nature. For more solitude, continue another 0.8 mile to smaller Chenamus Lake. Expect clouds of mosquitoes in July and early August. Cross the Columbia River on the Bridge of the Gods at Cascade Locks, go 6.1 miles east on Highway 14, then turn left and drive 0.9 mile to a junction in the town of Carson. Go straight, proceed 32.6 miles on Wind River Road and paved Forest Road 30, and then turn right on gravel Road 420 for 1.2 miles to the signed trailhead.

INDIAN RACETRACK

Round trip for loop: 8.2 miles / 1700 feet

A typically lovely meadow and pond in the southern Indian Heaven Wilderness with the added attraction of historical interest as this was the site of annual horse races by Native Americans until the 1920s. The place can be reached by several trails, but the most interesting is a loop from the south along the Pacific Crest Trail (PCT) that returns via Red Mountain Lookout (views!) and rough dirt Road 6048. Drive as in Trip 23 to the four-way junction on Road 65, but turn right (east) on gravel Road 60 and go 2 miles to the PCT crossing.

TRAPPER CREEK

Round trip to lower campsite: 6 miles / 900 feet (although the best waterfalls are farther upstream)

A heavily forested creek canyon with lots of small waterfalls and old-growth forests that is now protected as wilderness. The trail is ruggedly up and down, but it is open for most of the year and is a good option for a spring or fall hike. Cross the Columbia River on the Bridge of the Gods at Cascade Locks, go 6.1 miles east on Highway 14, then turn left and drive 0.9 mile to a junction in the town of Carson. Go straight, proceed 13.6 miles on Wind River Road, and then turn left on Mineral Springs Road. After 0.4 mile you turn right on gravel Road 5401 and proceed 0.4 mile to the trailhead.

Oregon Coast and Coast Range

BLOOM LAKE

Round trip: 2.7 miles / 450 feet

This relatively new and very convenient trail leads to a small lake with cutthroat trout fishing, beaver activity, pretty forests, and scenic skunk cabbage bogs. The trailhead is at a large road pullout near Milepost 24.5 on the south side of U.S. Highway 26.

SPRUCE RUN TRAIL TO LOST LAKE

Distance and elevation gains are not yet known.

As of 2008, this very promising trail was still under construction, but it will eventually provide some lovely creekside hiking and scenic access to a pretty lake with good campsites. Contact the Clatsop State Forest in Astoria (503-325-5451) for the latest information. Access will be off the Nehalem River Road south of its junction with U.S. Highway 26 west of Portland.

CENTRAL GALES CREEK TRAIL

Round trip to best camping area: 9 miles / 500 feet

A lovely and uncrowded creekside ramble along the upper reaches of Gales Creek amid lush Coast Range forest. The trail passes a couple of small waterfalls on side streams and offers the chance to see elk. Only mediocre camps are available, so you have to improvise a bit. Start from Gales Creek Campground just off State Highway 6 near Milepost 35.

Columbia River Gorge

PACIFIC COAST TRAIL SOUTH PAST TABLE MOUNTAIN

One way: 16.4 miles / 1500 feet (with lots of downhill)

Best done as a point-to-point, mostly downhill adventure, this route starts at the remote Three-Corner Rock Trailhead and follows the Pacific Crest Trail (PCT) along a magnificently scenic ridgeline (with one wildly scenic campsite) before descending to the Columbia River. The only water on the ridge is from a small spring that stops flowing around midsummer. May and June offer the best flower show. The lower trailhead is along Washington Highway 14 just east of North Bonneville. To reach the upper trailhead, start from Washougal along Highway 14 east of Vancouver and go 17.8 miles north and east on paved Washougal River Road. Turn right on gravel Road W2000, drive 10.6 miles to a junction at Rock Creek Pass, then take the second right and go 0.3 mile on a rocky road to the PCT crossing.

GILLETTE LAKE

Round trip: 5 miles / 450 feet

A low-elevation section of the PCT travels over a mostly forested, up-and-down landscape to an unspectacular but pleasant lake that is accessible nearly all year. You can continue the hike another 1.3 miles to a nice viewpoint at Greenleaf Overlook. The well-signed trailhead is just east of the town of North Bonneville along State Highway 14 on the Washington side of the Columbia River.

MULTNOMAH BASIN LOOP

Round trip for loop: 11.3 miles / 2950 feet

A scenic area of old-growth forest with a lovely meadow in the old glacial cirque on the north side of Larch Mountain. The most scenic approach is from Multnomah Falls on Interstate 84 with a hike past a string of waterfalls on Multnomah Creek. The trip is better if it is done as a loop with the view-packed Franklin Ridge Trail.

MOFFETT CREEK TRAIL

Round trip to small lake with campsites atop ridge: 19 miles / 3500 feet

A rough and little-used trail that connects Nesmith Point with Tanner Creek in a rarely visited section of the Gorge. The trail, which offers excellent and unusual views of Tanner Butte and rugged Mt. Talapus, also provides access to an abandoned trail to Wauneka Point with its Native American rock pits and superb views of the Columbia River. It is more scenic to approach from the east via Tanner Creek (see Trip 31 for directions). Walk the closed Tanner Creek Road for 5 miles, then turn west, ford the creek, and start a long, switchbacking climb.

BENSON PLATEAU

Round trip to best campsite at the headwaters of Ruckel Creek: 16 miles / 4150 feet

The goal is a remarkably flat forested plateau with lots of exploring and fine views of the peaks and canyons of the Columbia River Gorge. Getting there, unfortunately, requires a long, tough climb by any of several trails. The gentlest approach is via the Pacific Crest Trail from the north, which includes one excellent viewpoint along the way. See Trip 33 for driving directions and a map.

Mount Hood Area

DEVILS PEAK LOOKOUT

Round trip: 8 miles / 3200 feet

A long, tough, woodsy climb eventually leads to a grand viewpoint of Mt. Hood and an old lookout building that is available for overnight use on a first-come, first-served basis. A nearby spring provides water. Drive U.S. Highway 26 1.4 miles east of Zigzag, turn right on paved Still Creek Road, and right again after 0.1 mile at a confusing fork. Continue on pavement and good gravel another 3.3 miles to the obscure Cool Creek Trailhead. You can also reach the lookout via a much shorter trail from Kinzel Lake, but the access road is atrocious.

MIRROR LAKE

Round trip: 3.2 miles / 700 feet

An extremely popular hike to a lovely lake with postcard-perfect views of Mount Hood. Very crowded, so be prepared for plenty of company. Trail starts from a pullout off U.S. Highway 26 near Milepost 52 west of Government Camp.

WIND LAKE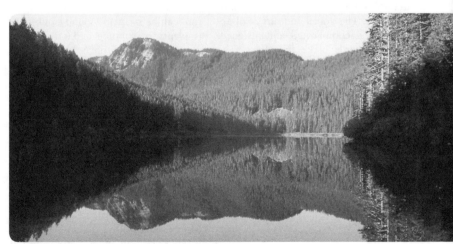
Round trip: 6.4 miles / 1400 feet

A shallow, forest-rimmed, and un-crowded lake on the south side of Tom Dick Mountain south of Mt. Hood. Start from the huge Ski Bowl West parking lot just west of Government Camp, follow rocky jeep roads and un-signed trails to the ridge at the top of the ski runs, and then hike west to the lake. Fishing is poor due to the shal-lowness of the lake.

Clackamas River Country

CLACKAMAS RIVER TRAIL
Round trip to the best campsite: 9.4 miles / 300 feet (with shorter and longer options)

A lovely hike along the clear Clacka-mas River passing spectacular Pup Creek Falls along the way. The trail is open nearly all year, but is immediately across the river from a highway, so the hike is not secluded. Drive 15 miles southeast of Estacada on State High-way 224, turn right on Road 54, and soon reach the developed trailhead on the other side of a large bridge.

SKOOKUM LAKE
Round trip: 6.2 miles / 1600 feet

Once popular but now rarely visited after floods permanently closed the nearest roads, this tiny, forest-rimmed lake features a fine campsite, solitude, and very good fishing. Now accessed by a scenic but hard to find trail that climbs over the shoulder of Thunder Mountain (good views), then switch-backs down to the lake. From Estacada go southeast 29.5 miles on State High-way 224, turn right on Road 63 for 3.4 miles, then right on Road 6320 for 1.3 miles. Turn sharply right on gravel Road 6322 for 6 miles, then go straight on Road 4620 and drive 3.1 miles to the unsigned trailhead on the right.

SILVER KING LAKE
Round trip: 10.8 miles / 1900 feet

A pretty little woodsy lake at the end of a scenic hike along Whetstone Ridge in the western Bull of the Woods Wil-derness. The ridge features some nice

Blue Lake, southern Mount Rainier and Goat Rocks area

vistas, although the lake is viewless. From Estacada go southeast 29.5 miles on State Highway 224, turn right on Road 63 for 3.6 miles, then right on Road 70 for 8.6 miles. Fork right onto gravel Road 7030 for 6.4 miles, and then turn right on a spur road to the trailhead.

WELCOME LAKES

Round trip: 9 miles / 1900 feet

A gentle woods walk past a waterfall on Elk Lake Creek, then a tough climb up to two small lakes in the Bull of the Woods Wilderness. The lower lake is prettier but the upper lake has better campsites. Follow directions for Trip 54, but instead of turning on Road 6340 go straight on Road 63 for 7 miles past several intersections to a fork at the end of pavement. Go right on Road 6380 and drive 2.9 miles to the Elk Lake Creek Trailhead.

BUTTE LAKES

Round trip: 1.8 miles / 200 feet

A group of small but very attractive lakes accessed by a short and easy trail in the Santiam State Forest southeast of Silverton. The gravel and dirt road access is long, complicated, and unsigned, so few people make the effort. The lakes provide pretty scenery and nice swimming. Start from Scotts Mills on Oregon Highway 213 with a good map (the best is *Salem District—Eastside* by the BLM) and a sense of adventure, then head southeast on Crooked Finger Road. The directions are far too complicated to detail, but it's about 25 miles to the blocked road at the unsigned trailhead on the right.

Mount Jefferson and Vicinity

OPAL CREEK

Round trip to camps at Cedar Flats: 10 miles / 550 feet

Magnificent old-growth forest and a wonderfully clear stream highlight this relatively easy hike in the Cascade Mountains west of Salem. Other noteworthy features include Jawbone Flats, an old mining settlement now used as a nature learning center, and several waterfalls. The trail follows a jeep road into Jawbone Flats, and then an up-and-down trail south along gorgeous Opal Creek. From Salem, drive 22 miles east on Highway 22 to Mehama, then turn left on Little North Fork Road and go 15.5 miles to the end of pavement. Continue on bumpy gravel Road 2209 for 5.6 miles to the trailhead where the road is gated.

OPAL LAKE

Round trip: 1.2 miles / 350 feet

A deep, meadow- and forest-rimmed lake at the end of a downhill trail in a remote area north of Detroit Reservoir. The lake has no views and the access trail can be steep and muddy, but there is plenty of solitude and nice fishing for brook trout. From Salem, drive 50 miles east on Highway 22 to a junction just before the bridge near Detroit. Turn left (north) here on one-lane paved French Creek Road (Road 2233), go 4.2 miles, and then turn right on gravel Road 2207. Follow this narrow road for 5.9 miles to the trailhead.

MARION LAKE

Round trip: 6 miles / 800 feet

A gentle, uphill trail in the southern Mount Jefferson Wilderness past lovely Lake Ann and a pretty waterfall takes you up to huge Marion Lake. The trip has been a favorite for generations of outdoor lovers. Sadly, this area was badly burned in the 2003 B&B Complex Fire, so it is now mostly a shadeless sea of blackened snags. Expect lots of mosquitoes in July. From Salem, drive 65 miles east on Oregon Highway 22 to Marion Forks, turn left (east) on Marion Creek Road (Forest Road 2255), and go 5.5 miles to the road-end trailhead.

PARISH LAKE

Round trip: 1 mile / 250 feet

An easy hike into a small, forest-rimmed lake in the Western Cascades with decent views of the nearby Three Pyramids. The lake is rarely crowded and has good fishing for brook trout. From Salem, drive 76 miles east on Oregon Highway 22, turn right (west) on initially paved then gravel Forest Road 2266 for 5 miles to the trailhead.

GORDON LAKES

Round trip: 0.8 mile / 175 feet

A short and easy downhill stroll into a pair of scenic little lakes beneath the impressive cliffs of Soapgrass Mountain in the Western Cascades. The area is little known and rarely visited. The nearby meadows are great for wild-flowers from late June through mid-July, while the lakes offer decent fishing for cutthroat trout and fine swimming. Take Interstate 5 south to Albany Exit 233, and then take U.S. Highway 20 east to a junction 28 miles past Sweet Home. Turn south at a sign for House Rock Campground onto gravel Forest Road 2044, drive 5.5 miles, then go right on Road 230 for 2.6 miles to the road-end trailhead.

PATJENS LAKES

Round trip for loop: 6.1 miles / 450 feet

A very popular loop trail past a string of pretty lakes in the northern Mount Washington Wilderness. Campsites are only mediocre, but the views of Mt. Washington, especially over Middle Patjens Lake, are excellent. Expect lots of dayhikers, mosquitoes in July, and countless thousands of frogs. From Salem, drive 89 miles east on State Highway 22 and U.S. Highway 20 to a junction just before Santiam Pass. Turn south on Big Lake Road and drive 4 miles, staying on the main paved road past Hoodoo Ski Area and Big Lake Campground to the trailhead on the right.

ROCKPILE LAKE

Round trip: 11.8 miles / 1400 feet

A pretty but fishless pond along the Pacific Crest Trail (PCT) north of Three Fingered Jack. The basin immediately around this scenic little lake was not damaged in the 2003 B&B Complex Fire, but much of the access trail was badly scorched. The lake can be reached either by a little traveled loop trail from the east or along the PCT past Wasco Lake from south. The southern approach has better views of Three Fingered Jack and somewhat less fire damage. For the south approach, start from Santiam Pass, go east 7.6 miles on U.S. Highway 20, then turn left on paved Jack Lake Road (Forest Road 12). Follow this road for 4.4 miles, turn left on Road 1230 for 1.8 miles, and then left on gravel Road 1234 and proceed 5 miles to the Jack Lake Trailhead.

APPENDIX B
Recommended Reading

Even the briefest glance at the outdoor section of any local bookstore shows that there is a lot of interest from the reading public in the Pacific Northwest outdoors. It is also clear that owning all of the available volumes would be overkill in the extreme. Here are some of the author's favorites to help you build your own outdoor library.

This book is designed for those seeking shorter, one-night backpacking trips. If you prefer dayhiking, the two best guides for the Portland area are this author's own *Afoot & Afield Portland/Vancouver* (Wilderness Press, 2nd ed., 2008), which covers literally every trail within an hour's drive of the Portland area, and *100 Hikes in Northwest Oregon* by William L. Sullivan (Navillus Press, 2006), which is less comprehensive, but covers many fine trails within a 2 hours' drive of the city.

Once you have moved beyond the weekend trip and want to tackle a longer backpacking adventure, pick up copies of this author's *Backpacking Oregon, Backpacking Washington,* and *Backpacking Idaho* (Wilderness Press), which detail the best 3- to 10-day backpacking vacations in every corner of their respective states.

For proof that the benefits of taking your kids hiking considerably outweigh the extra time and effort involved, read *Last Child in the Woods: Saving Our Children from Nature-Deficit Disorder* by Richard Louv (Algonquin Books, 2005). It should be required reading for every American parent. For more on the how-to side of things for outdoor travel with children, two good resources are *Camping and Backpacking with Children* by Steven Boga (Stackpole Books, 1995) and *Extreme Kids* by Scott Graham (Wilderness Press, 2006). You might also consider picking up a copy of a fun little book designed for evening entertainment entitled *Spooky Campfire Tales* by S. E. Schlosser (Globe Pequot Press, 2007).

Some of the better books on the various aspects of backpacking are *Backpacker Magazine's Everyday Wisdom* series, which cover a wide range of topics with hundreds of useful tips from outdoor experts. *Leave No Trace: A Guide to New Wilderness Etiquette* (Mountaineers Books, 2nd ed., 2003) is particularly useful. An excellent single volume guide for the sport of backpacking is *The Backpacker's Field Manual: A Comprehensive Guide to Mastering Backcountry Skills* by Rick Curtis (Three Rivers Press, 1998).

Two classic tomes that cover the topic even more thoroughly are *The Complete Walker IV* by Colin Fletcher and Chip Rawlins (Alfred A. Knopf, 2002), and *Mountaineering: The Freedom of the Hills* by Steven M. Cox and Kris Fulsaas (Mountaineers Books, 1997).

Three other good books you might consider are *The Ultralight Backpacker* by Ryel Kestenbaum (McGraw-Hill Professional, 2001), which goes a bit overboard, in my opinion, on the ultralight craze, but still has lots of good ideas; *Basic Essentials: Wilderness First Aid* by William Forgey, M.D. (Falcon, 2nd ed., 1999); and *Mountain Weather: Backcountry Forecasting and Weather Safety for Hikers, Campers, Climb-*

ers, Skiers, and Snowboarders by Jeff Renner (Mountaineers Books, 2005).

There are a number of excellent books for hikers interested in the natural history of the Pacific Northwest. The best local wildflower guide for amateurs is *Wildflowers of the Pacific Northwest* by Mark Turner and Phyllis Gustafson (Timber Press, 2006). The maps are confusing and the index is hard to use, but the book is otherwise superb. If you are interested in birds, the best general guide is The National Geographic Society's *Field Guide to the Birds of North America* (National Geographic, 5th ed., 2006). A particularly fun and interesting little book on our avian friends is *Why Woodpeckers Don't Get Headaches, And Other Bird Questions You Know You Want to Ask* by Mike O'Conner (Beacon Press, 2007). Two useful books for those interested in edible plants are *Field Guide to Edible Wild Plants* by Bradford Angier (Stackpole Books, 1974), and *Northwest Foraging* by Doug Benoliel (Signpost Books, 1974). The best one-volume general natural history guide to our area, which covers all the most common trees, shrubs, mammals, amphibians, and reptiles, is *The Audubon Society Nature Guide: Western Forests* (Alfred A. Knopf, 1990). Lastly, for hikers interested in the geology of the Cascade Mountains, a copy of *Fire & Ice: The Cascade Volcanoes* by Stephen L. Harris (Harcourt, 1987) is a must.

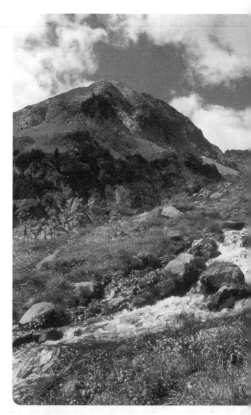

Pyramid Peak over Pyramid Park, Mount Rainier National Park (Trip 5)

Finally, for general entertainment on the trail, every hiker should read *A Walk in the Woods* by Bill Bryson (Broadway, 1999). Not reading this book is a disservice to your funny bone.

APPENDIX C

Conservation Organizations and Outdoor Clubs

Friends of the Columbia Gorge
522 S.W. 5th Avenue, Suite 720
Portland, OR 97204
(503) 241-3762
www.gorgefriends.org

The Mazamas
527 S.E. 43rd Avenue
Portland, OR 97215
(503) 227-2345
www.mazamas.org

Oregon Chapter Sierra Club
2950 S.E. Stark Street, Suite 110
Portland, OR 97214
(503) 238-0442
www.oregon.sierraclub.org

The Nature Conservancy of Oregon
821 S.E. 14th Avenue
Portland, OR 97214
(503) 802-8100
www.nature.org/states/oregon

Portland Audubon Society
5151 Cornell Road
Portland, OR 97210
(503) 292-6855
www.audubonportland.org

Trails Club of Oregon
P.O. Box 1243
Portland, OR 97207
(503) 233-2740
www.trailsclub.org

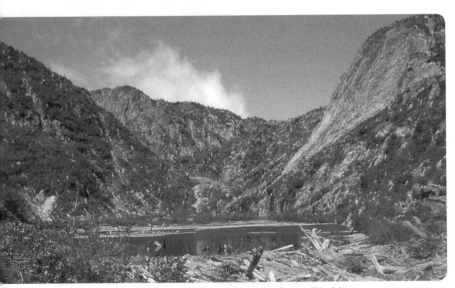

Grizzly Lake, Mount Saint Helens National Volcanic Monument (Trip 14)

APPENDIX D
Land Agencies and Information Sources

Bureau of Land Management:
Salem District
1717 Fabry Road S.E.
Salem, OR 97306
(503) 375-5646
www.blm.gov/or/districts/salem

Clatsop State Forest
92219 Highway 202
Astoria, OR 97103
(503) 325-5451
www.oregon.gov/odf/field/astoria

Columbia River Gorge
National Scenic Area
902 Wasco Avenue, Suite 200
Hood River, OR 97031
(541) 308-1700
www.fs.fed.us/r6/columbia

Deschutes National Forest
www.fs.fed.us/r6/centraloregon

Sisters Ranger District
P.O. Box 249
Sisters, OR 97759
(541) 549-7700

Deschutes River State Recreation Area
89600 Biggs-Rufus Highway
Wasco, OR 97065
(541) 739-2322, ext. 0

Ecola State Park and
Oswald West State Park
Both managed by:
Nehalem Bay State Park
P.O. Box 366
Nehalem, OR 97131
(503) 368-5943

Gifford Pinchot National Forest
www.fs.fed.us/gpnf

Cowlitz Valley Ranger District
10024 U.S. Highway 12
P.O. Box 670
Randle, WA 98377
(360) 497-1100

Mount Adams Ranger District
2455 Highway 141
Trout Lake, WA 98650
(509) 395-3400

Mount Hood National Forest
www.fs.fed.us/r6/mthood

Barlow Ranger District
780 N.E. Court Street
Dufur, OR 97021
(541) 467-2291

Clackamas River Ranger District
595 N.W. Industrial Way
Estacada, OR 97023
(503) 630-6861

Hood River Ranger District
6780 Oregon Highway 35
Mount Hood-Parkdale, OR 97041
(541) 352-6002

Zigzag Ranger District
70220 East Highway 26
Zigzag, OR 97049
(503) 622-3191

Mount Rainier National Park
Wilderness Information Center
55210 238th Avenue East
Ashford, WA 98376
(360) 569-2211, ext. 3314
www.nps.gov/mora/

Mount St. Helens National
Volcanic Monument
42218 N.E. Yale Bridge Road
Amboy, WA 98601
(360) 449-7800
www.fs.fed.us/gpnf/mshnvm/

Nature of the Northwest
Information Center
800 N. Oregon Street, Suite 177
Portland, OR 97232
(503) 872-2752
www.naturenw.org

Olympic National Forest
www.fs.fed.us/r6/olympic/

Hood Canal Ranger District
295142 Highway 101 South
P.O. Box 280
Quilcene, WA 98376
(360) 765-2200

Olympic National Park
Wilderness Information Center
600 E. Park Avenue
Port Angeles, WA 98382
(360) 565-3100
www.nps.gov/olym/

Oregon State Parks
725 Summer Street N.E., Suite C
Salem, OR 97301
(800) 551-6949
www.oregonstateparks.org

North Coast Field Office
4157 N. U.S. Highway 101, Suite 127
Lincoln City, OR 97367
(503) 994-8152

Tillamook State Forest
www.oregon.gov/ODF/TSF

Forest Grove District Office
801 Gales Creek Road
Forest Grove, OR 97116
(503) 357-2191

Wenatchee National Forest
www.fs.fed/r6/wenatchee

Naches Ranger District
10237 Highway 12
Naches, WA 98937
(509) 653-1400

Willamette National Forest
www.fs.fed.us/r6/willamette

Detroit Ranger District
HC 73, Box 320
Mill City, OR 97360
(503) 854-3366

McKenzie River Ranger District
57600 McKenzie Highway
McKenzie Bridge, OR 97413
(541) 822-3381

Yakama Nation
Department of Natural Resources
P.O. Box 151
Toppenish, WA 98948
(509) 865-5121, ext. 4653

Index

About the Author

Douglas Lorain's family moved to the Pacific Northwest in 1969, and he has been obsessively hitting the trails of his home region ever since. With the good fortune to grow up in an outdoor-oriented family, he has vivid memories of countless camping, biking, birdwatching, and other trips in every corner of this spectacular area. Over the years he calculates that he has logged well over 30,000 trail miles in this corner of the continent, and despite a history that includes being bitten by a rattlesnake, shot at by a hunter, charged by grizzly bears (twice!), and donating countless gallons of blood to "invertebrate vampires," he happily sees no end in sight.

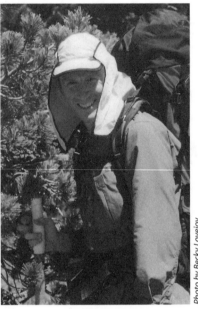

Photo by Becky Lovejoy

Lorain is a photographer and recipient of the National Outdoor Book Award. His books cover only the best trips from the thousands of hikes and backpacking trips he has taken throughout Oregon, Washington, and Idaho. His photographs have been featured in numerous magazines, calendars, and books, and his other guidebook titles include *100 Classic Hikes in Oregon, Backpacking Idaho, Backpacking Oregon, Backpacking Washington,* and *Afoot & Afield Portland/Vancouver.*

Although he considers his real home to be on the trail, those few days he is forced to spend indoors, he lives in Portland, Oregon, with his wife, Becky Lovejoy.